THE BIRTH BOOK

THE BIRTH BOOK

An OB-GYN's Guide to Demystifying Labor and Delivery

DR. JENNIFER LINCOLN

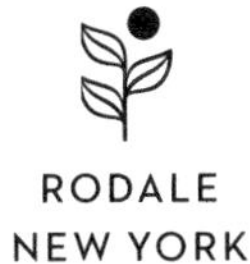

RODALE
NEW YORK

Rodale Books
An imprint of Random House
A division of Penguin Random House LLC
1745 Broadway, New York, NY 10019
rodalebooks.com | randomhousebooks.com
penguinrandomhouse.com

A Rodale Trade Paperback Original

This book does not serve as a replacement for professional or medical advice or treatment. Readers should regularly consult medical professionals in matters relating to health and particularly with respect to any symptoms that may require diagnosis or medical attention.

This book does not constitute a doctor–patient relationship. All opinions are the author's own and do not represent her employers or any organizations to which she belongs.

ISBN 978-0-593-98050-7
Ebook ISBN 978-0-593-98051-4

Printed in the United States of America on acid-free paper

2nd Printing

Book Team: Production editor: Cassie Gitkin • Managing editor: Allison Fox
Production manager: Maggie Hart • Copy editor: Sue Warga • Indexer: Gina Guilinger
Proofreaders: Cyrus Chin, Rachael Clements, Pam Feinstein, Andrea Gordon, Ella Maoz

The authorized representative in the EU for product safety and compliance is Penguin Random House Ireland, Morrison Chambers, 32 Nassau Street, Dublin D02 YH68, Ireland. **https://eu-contact.penguin.ie**

For every patient I have had or will have the privilege of caring for: You all teach me more than any book ever could. Thank you.

For those of you I get to work alongside, who run toward the fire instead of away from it (even during a full moon): I am so lucky to work with and learn from such caring, dedicated professionals.

For anyone who has ever experienced a loss or a traumatic birth, or who was not able to get the respectful care you deserved because of your zip code, your race, your social status, or our broken system: Know that I will keep fighting and advocating for you.

CONTENTS

IS IT TIME?

WELCOME TO THE (BIRTHDAY) PARTY

THE GRAND ENTRANCE (OR EXIT)

STILLBIRTH

INTRODUCTION

Birth sure is . . . something.

It can be planned and empowering and fun and defining and joyful.

It can also be chaotic and unexpected and painful and disrespectful and traumatic.

So what's someone to do when they're pregnant and trying to prepare for what might be one of the best days of their life, but they've heard the horror stories and seen the social media posts and know the stats about giving birth in America?

When their prenatal visits last fifteen minutes? And when more than half of U.S. counties lack a hospital with a labor and delivery unit?

How do you get the birth you want and deserve, especially when you might not even know what you're entitled to and what you could be asking for?

As a board-certified OB-GYN practicing as an OB hospitalist, I have years of experience in seeing how we get birth right—and how we can do so much better. Time and time again I see my patients coming into the hospital not knowing what to expect, and not even knowing where to begin in asking how to get what they have every right to: a respectful, individualized, evidence-based birth experience.

Let me be clear that this is *not* their failure—it's ours.

Our country has never been set up to help pregnant people be fully informed about birth. Our prenatal visits are too short. Our medical practices are too inconsistent. Our hierarchy is too rigid. Our schools are too restricted when it comes to laying the groundwork for understanding our bodies. Our systems are too racist and classist. And our for-profit healthcare industry is too corrupt, which is at the core of many (but not all) of the problems I just described.

If you're reading this, pregnant and preparing to have your baby, I don't want the above to frighten you. Instead, I want you to know that **you absolutely can rise above all these barriers and get the birth experience you've dreamed of.** It starts with being educated—because once you know what you can ask for, you are taking the first step in being empowered to get it.

That's why I wrote this book: to help level the playing field. You deserve to get your questions answered . . . and to even know what questions you can ask. Until now, a book that focuses only on the birth experience written by an OB-GYN who does this for a living hasn't existed. My expertise, coupled with the understanding that there is rarely one way to do things, will (hopefully) make for an easy-to-understand guide so you can get the birth you want and deserve.

I also acknowledge the reality that is healthcare in America: Access to some of the things I discuss in my book may be limited based on where you are, or what kind of insurance you might have. Your income or ethnicity or zip code should not matter when having a baby, and yet I would be lying if I didn't say it sometimes does. I know not everything I mention in this book will be an option for you, and that is *wrong*. Yet I still want you to be able to go in fully informed—and maybe even one day advocate to help us make some lasting change in this country.

I recommend that you use this book as you see fit: You can read it cover-to-cover or only focus on what matters most to you. It's OK to skip over sections that might stress you out or make you worry more. I do want to highlight that while the book has a section on stillbirth, there is some mention of it throughout other sections as well.

A quick note on language: I will use the terms "pregnant woman," "pregnant person," "birthing person," "mother," "father," "parent," and "partner" interchangeably throughout this book. That is because these are terms my readers will use to describe themselves, and I want *everyone* to see themselves here. If it feels uncomfortable to you to hear the term "pregnant person," I ask you to understand it is not about erasing anyone but rather about including more people. I write this as a mother myself, who knows she is still a mom even when the literature uses more inclusive terms.

Finally, for any doctor or midwife who is reading this and is worrying I'm making your practices more difficult by pulling back the curtain on what we do, I'd ask you to take a moment and reframe what an informed patient is and means to us. I know I love it when my patients ask me about a procedure or something they saw online, because it means they feel they can speak up, they're informed, and they want to be an active participant in the labor process—not a bother or an adversary, but rather a true partner in a very intimate process. How could we not want that?

I hope this book leaves you informed and empowered to know you are worthy of having the birth experience you want and deserve.

Dr. Jennifer Lincoln

THE WHO AND THE WHERE

FROM BIRTH CENTER TO HOSPITAL IN THE MIDDLE OF THE NIGHT

My pager went off at 2 A.M., and I immediately recognized the number. It was a midwife from the local birth center—they had a woman in labor who needed to be transferred to my hospital.

I learned that she'd been in labor for days and was exhausted. Her cervix was 6 centimeters dilated but hadn't changed over the past ten hours. She was sad at needing to leave her birth center and had a huge fear of hospitals after losing her dad one year prior. Basically, she had zero desire to meet me, and her feelings weren't subtle.

The midwife and I finished our conversation, and I left my call room to go chat with the labor nurse who would be caring for this patient. When I saw who it would be I smiled, because I knew this was the exact right person to help ease this mom's transition into a situation that felt scary and unwanted.

I've always been proud of how my group has cared for people transferring from home or birth centers, but I'd be lying if I said that my mind didn't always contemplate the worst-case scenarios before such people arrived. What if she had an infection or hemorrhaged from being in labor so long? How was her baby doing? What if her baby was breech and no one noticed? If she needed a C-section, would she be open to it? How difficult would it be to build rapport?

Our patient arrived an hour later, not ready to talk to me because she was in so much pain and so exhausted. We prioritized comfort, and she received an epidural and slept hard for a few hours. When she (and her partner) woke up, I introduced myself. We talked about her goals, and I clarified that her main one was to avoid a C-section. Her nurse and I discussed why I recommended starting Pitocin to try to help move her labor along, and as a way to actually get her the vaginal birth she so badly wanted. We reviewed risks and alternatives. We acknowledged that we knew this wasn't her plan, but we would do everything we could to support them as this birth experience took a detour.

There was some crying, but also some laughing as we joked about comparing the hospital décor and linen quality to those of her birth center. At one point she said, "My midwife said you guys were nice, but I didn't really believe her. You guys are great, though."

In the end, she birthed a gorgeous baby boy who weighed almost nine pounds and had a ton of hair. There was some extra bleeding, but nothing we couldn't manage. She went home two days later, healthy and happy—though I am sure still carrying some trauma from not having the experience she had wished for. But I do hope her feeling seen and valued helped, even just a little bit.

WHERE CAN I HAVE MY BABY?

Technically, you can have your baby anywhere you want (well, maybe not anywhere)—but what I mean is that the answer doesn't always have to be a hospital. You might be surprised that an OB-GYN is starting her book with that statement, but my goal is to go beyond what we're always told—because that hasn't really worked well—and to meet people where they're at so that they can make informed, empowered decisions.

So yes, you can even choose to have your baby without any medical professionals around (called freebirthing or unassisted birth, this is the practice of having a baby on your own and sometimes includes forgoing prenatal care as well). That may sound out there, and as a hospital-based OB-GYN of course I have thoughts on it, but at the end of the day where you birth is your choice. However, we need to talk about the risks and benefits of all possible scenarios.

Community birth is a term that refers to a planned birth at home or in a birth center. You'll see me refer to that often, so I wanted to define it for you.

Here are common places you can choose to give birth, with my thoughts on each:

	What it is	Pros	Cons	Dr. Jen's notes
Hospital	What it sounds like! This is our most common model of birth in the United States.	• Access to pain medication options like an epidural and IV medications • Access to emergency care and specialists if needed • Nothing you need to do to prepare your home • Often covered by insurance • Tends to be more socially acceptable to many people	• Requires driving to it (this can be an issue if one isn't close by) • Higher rates of interventions like C-sections • A more medicalized feeling • You may see providers you don't know • Cost concerns are real	Many hospitals employ certified nurse midwives and have access to things like whirlpool baths for labor or even for waterbirths. If you're interested in this, it's important to ask early on in pregnancy to make sure your intended hospital has these resources available.

	What it is	Pros	Cons	Dr. Jen's notes
Home	Birthing at home, often with the oversight of a midwife (more on page 11 about the different types of midwives).	· No need to leave the comfort of your own home · Lower rates of interventions · Some midwives may offer nitrous oxide for pain relief · Can be more affordable than hospital birth · Helpful if you have other children and you don't have childcare, since you aren't leaving them · Often a combination of office and home visits prenatally, and often more postpartum visits than if you delivered with an OB-GYN in a hospital	· Requires preparation, including getting supplies · Lack of access to IV pain medications or epidurals · It still may require hospital transfer, which can result in a disjointed-feeling experience · Some emergencies happen too quickly for a hospital transfer, leading to potential life-threatening outcomes · May not be covered by insurance in some states	I want to note that a homebirth with an experienced midwife is very different from an unassisted freebirth at home. More on this in the coming pages.
Freestanding birth center	This is a birth center that may be run by a community or by certified nurse midwives. Care, delivery, and postpartum recovery can often happen in the same place.	Similar benefits as homebirth, but without having to prepare your own home	· Often the same as a homebirth · Have to get in a car to go somewhere	· Same safety profile as with homebirth · If you live far from a hospital but a birth center is closer to home, this can be a nice option.

	What it is	Pros	Cons	Dr. Jen's notes
Hospital-based birth center	A birth center that is co-located or nested within, but technically separate from, the hospital's labor and delivery unit.	Feels like a birth center but with access to all emergency care and resources that are on Labor and Delivery	• Unfortunately, not that common in the United States. • Can still have some of the medicalized drawbacks of a hospital birth (more interventions).	I wish we had this in every hospital!

TRANSFERRING INTO A HOSPITAL

Between 5 and 35 percent of all people who opt for a birth outside the hospital will need to transfer into one either during or after birth, with most situations being non-urgent. This is a huge range, but in general the rate is lower for those who've given birth vaginally before. Common reasons to transfer include wanting pain medication and stalled labor. For more, see page 178, "I planned a homebirth and have to transfer in; what should I know?"

I also think having an idea of *actual* numbers can be helpful in deciding where to have your baby. As you can see on the next page, planned homebirths, birth center births, and hospital births are associated with their own unique risks. It's up to you—ideally in consultation with a medical provider who understands the intricacies of your own health and pregnancy—to decide which of these risks are more acceptable to you and which are not.

	Planned birth at home or at a birth center (per 1,000 births)	**Planned hospital birth (per 1,000 births)**
Newborn seizures	1.3	0.4
Stillbirth and newborn death	3.9	1.8
Stillbirth if having a trial of labor after cesarean (TOLAC)	2.9	0.13
Severe tearing	9	13
Delivery by C-section	53	247
Labor induction	48	304
Blood transfusion	6	4

Whether or not you choose to have your baby in a hospital or at home is a personal decision, but I wouldn't be an OB-GYN if I didn't say that certain pregnancies are higher risk and can make a community birth a riskier event. Though rare, there are also some obstetric emergencies that can occur suddenly in even the lowest-risk pregnancy where not being in a hospital could be catastrophic. The flip side of the coin is that I readily acknowledge that hospital-based births are not perfect, and we have work to do to make our patients feel as supported as they may feel at home with a midwife.

If you have a pregnancy complicated by high blood pressure, a prior C-section, twins (or more), certain medical conditions, or a history of postpartum hemorrhage, shoulder dystocia, or other concerns, a hospital birth is likely safer for you and your baby. If any of these apply to you, it's important to have a good conversation with your doctor or midwife about your specific scenario, and to understand if they advise against a community birth.

My OB-GYN take-home point after all the above? Community births can **be done safely, and one of the best ways to achieve that is**

for the appropriate risk stratification for pregnancies that are low- versus high-risk. Ultimately, no one can force you to deliver in a hospital, but we tend to see worse outcomes when births that carried too many risks for a home or birth center birth were attempted in those places, with sometimes heartbreaking results.

KNOW THE LAWS

FOR HOMEBIRTHS

The laws on who midwives and doctors can care for out of the hospital vary by state. Certain pregnancy issues will be considered too risky for a birth center birth under one state's law but not another's, so ask your team what's the deal in your state.

FOR BIRTH CENTERS

Depending on if they are licensed by the state or federally, all birth centers will have regulations regarding who they can or cannot accept as a client. Ask your birth center team for details on what they can care for and for which complications they must refer patients elsewhere.

WHO CAN HELP ME DELIVER MY BABY?

It's not just we OB-GYNs who deliver babies! Of course, being one myself, I love being at births, but I also recognize that sometimes I am not needed. And the hard truth is that sometimes our field contributes to overusing interventions and not respecting the natural process of birth, which is why some people would rather not have an

OB-GYN at their delivery. Acknowledging this doesn't discredit what we bring to the table, but it does go a long way toward rebuilding trust and acknowledging that birth is a team sport.

Here's a description of the different providers who can be there with you on your baby's birthday—and while I know that not everyone has access to all these options, knowing what's out there can help guide you when you're deciding who to call after you get that positive pregnancy test:

Type of provider	Training	Pros	Potential cons
OB-GYNs	Four years of medical school, four years of OB-GYN residency (specialty training), passing of national certifying exam, annual required maintenance of certification	· They can handle complications and higher-risk pregnancies · Experts in C-sections and other interventions that may be needed · Insurance coverage is usually the standard	· Potential for increased interventions, as we don't always view birth through the same lens as midwives · Almost never available for homebirths
High-risk OB-GYNs (maternal-fetal medicine doctors or perinatologists)	Same as above, plus an additional three-year fellowship in high-risk obstetrics and ultrasound	· These doctors see the highest-risk patients · They may manage your entire prenatal care, or work in consultation with your OB-GYN or midwife	· Many provide prenatal care but don't do deliveries, so you may not know the doctor who will be at your birth · Potential for increased interventions

Type of provider	Training	Pros	Potential cons
Family medicine doctors	Four years of medical school, three years of family medicine residency (many who do prenatal care and deliveries do additional training in obstetrics), passing of national certifying exam, annual required maintenance of certification	• Can manage low-risk pregnancies • Can continue to be your doctor *and* your baby's and entire family's doctor, so excellent continuity of care	• Most don't do C-sections, so a transfer of care would be necessary in that scenario • Not able to manage high-risk pregnancies or birth, necessitating transfer of care • Tend to be regional (i.e., rural areas, West Coast)
Certified nurse midwives (CNMs) or certified midwives (CMs)	Complete accredited graduate-level midwifery program, passed a national certifying exam for licensure, required ongoing maintenance of certification *(Note: CNMs are also registered nurses)*	• CNMs are licensed and can prescribe in all states • Practice in all settings (home, birth center, hospitals) • Have lower rates of interventions like C-sections and epidural use • Often view birth as more of a physiologic, or more natural, process • May be able to provide prenatal/postnatal care at home	• Not able to manage high-risk pregnancies or birth, which may mean transfer of care during pregnancy or labor • CM licensing, ability to prescribe, and insurance coverage are limited (state-dependent)

Type of provider	Training	Pros	Potential cons
Certified professional midwives (CPMs)	• High school education or equivalent required, as well as graduation from an accredited program or self-study portfolio evaluation • Apprenticeship process with a qualified preceptor • Satisfy clinical requirements (such as a certain number of documented births, prenatal/postnatal exams, certification in CPR and neonatal resuscitation) and pass a national certifying exam (the North American Registry of Midwives oversees this certification process)	• Practice in homes and birth centers • Have lower rates of interventions • Often view birth as more of a physiologic, or natural, process • Focus on individualized care • Can provide prenatal/ postnatal care at home	• Not able to manage high-risk pregnancies or birth, necessitating transfer of care • Not available for hospital births • Not able to write prescriptions • Scope of practice and insurance coverage vary by state
Direct entry midwives (DEMs), also called registered midwives (RMs) or licensed midwives (LMs)	Apprenticeship, self-study, midwifery school, or a college-based program, all distinct from nursing		• These terms can be confusing, as what they mean varies by state • Not able to manage high-risk pregnancies or birth, necessitating transfer of care • Not available for hospital births • May be able to write prescriptions (state-dependent) • Limited licensing, and what is required for licensing varies by state—be sure to ask your midwife about this

Type of provider	Training	Pros	Potential cons
Community/traditional/lay midwives	Unlicensed midwives who have informal education via apprenticeship models or have formal training but may not be licensed or credentialed. Training can vary.	• Often experts in their communities and cultures, and view birth through the lens of their religion or cultural practices • May be the only accessible providers in some rural or isolated communities • Offer homebirths and prenatal/postnatal care	• No standardization of training or practice regulation • Are not able to prescribe or carry many emergency medications that may be needed in labor • Not covered by most insurances
Naturopathic physician midwife	Four years of naturopathic medical school, completion of midwifery training under a licensed naturopathic midwife, passing a national board exam	• Practice in homes and birth centers • May be able to provide prenatal/postnatal care at home • Many often provide care for babies and families as well	• Licensed/regulated in twenty-three states and the District of Columbia • The field of naturopathic medicine is not without its controversies and variations in training
Yourself (freebirth, unassisted birth)	Some people participate in online groups or training to prepare for birth; many forgo any prenatal care	• Birth in the comfort of your own home • No medical bills (if no complications arise) • Many say it feels more natural and empowering	• Lack of trained medical professionals in emergencies can be catastrophic or fatal

If it feels confusing to try to understand the differences between different types of midwives, that's because it is. States vary so much in terms of licensing and laws, and midwives can vary in how they advertise their credentials. If you are considering using a midwife for a community birth, I highly recommend the following:

1. Check with your state's medical board to see what is allowed in your state (i.e., can those midwives prescribe or carry lifesaving medications, etc.).
2. For CNMs or CMs: You can verify your midwife's credentials at the American Midwifery Certification Board (page 297).
3. For state licensure of a midwife: You can go to your state medical board's page (page 297) to do a license inquiry search.
4. For CPMs: You can make an inquiry at the North American Registry of Midwives by emailing support@narm.org.

I'VE CHOSEN A HOSPITAL— WHAT SHOULD I ASK ABOUT?

I want to preface this section by acknowledging that not everyone has the luxury of being able to choose among multiple hospitals for birthing—but even if you don't, asking these questions can still be helpful so that you know what to expect and are prepared on your big day.

Many of these questions can be answered on a hospital's website, so you might want to start there. Your OB-GYN or midwife will also be able to answer quite a few, or you can call the hospital's labor and delivery unit and ask to speak with the charge nurse or nurse manager.

Don't feel obligated to ask all these questions if they don't pertain to you or aren't important to you, though—and definitely add in anything else you might want to know!

1. Does my insurance cover this hospital? And everyone who works in it?
2. Can you care for my baby if they are born preterm? Or is there a gestational age cutoff below which you'd have to transfer my baby to a different hospital?
3. Are an anesthesiologist and operating room team available and physically present in the hospital 24/7?
4. Is the anesthesiologist employed by the hospital? Do they take my insurance? Or is it a separate contracted group?
5. What is the C-section rate for the hospital?
6. Do you offer doulas? If not, am I able to have my own doula present?
7. Does the hospital have a blood bank that carries all blood products, or only some?
8. Am I able to donate my baby's cord blood to a public bank?
9. If I want to take home my placenta, is that going to be an issue?
10. What are my options for pain relief besides an epidural, such as nitrous oxide?
11. Are midwives present on Labor and Delivery, and how do they work with the physicians?
12. Does the hospital offer tours and/or birth and breastfeeding prep classes?
13. Can my pediatrician see my baby in the hospital, or does a hospital-employed pediatrician care for all babies?

14. Do you offer tubs or whirlpool baths for laboring in? How likely is it that one will be available for me to use?

15. Is waterbirth an option?

16. Is wireless fetal monitoring an option?

17. Is an OB hospitalist present on the unit 24/7?

18. If I have a C-section, am I able to do skin-to-skin in the operating room?

19. What is the visitor policy?

20. Is this a designated baby-friendly hospital?

21. What breastfeeding help is available to me?

22. Do babies room in (stay in the room with you), and if so, is there a respite nursery if I need a break?

23. What is the hospital's policy on the timing of newborn baths?

24. Is there access to donor milk if I need to supplement, and if so, is it available for anyone or reserved for certain babies, such as those in the neonatal intensive care unit (NICU)?

25. Am I able to get comprehensive reproductive care, such as an abortion if needed or a tubal ligation after I have my baby, or are there religious restrictions?

I know it might seem like a lot of questions. But who wants to arrive at their chosen hospital in active labor, only to find out that their top priority (laboring in a tub, for instance) isn't even an option? I've seen these disappointments happen before, and I want to help you avoid that experience by being prepared.

HOW DO I PICK AN OB-GYN OR HOSPITAL MIDWIFE?

OK, you've opted to birth in a hospital—but how the heck do you pick the person who's going to be there throughout your pregnancy and at your birth?

WHAT TO ASK YOUR DOCTOR/MIDWIFE PRENATALLY

- Do you take my insurance?
- What hospital(s) do you deliver babies at?
- How do I get in touch with you after hours/on weekends?
- Is there an online portal for questions/results/scheduling?
- Are there males in the practice (*if this matters to you*)?
- Will I see medical students, midwifery students, residents, or other learners?
- Do you partner with midwives?
- Are you OK with me having a doula?
- Who can I expect to see in the hospital and at my birth?
- Is there an OB hospitalist present 24/7 on Labor and Delivery?
- Can I take photos? Video?
- What is your C-section rate? Episiotomy rate?
- If I need a C-section:
    - Can my support person be in the operating room with me?
    - Will you use a clear drape so I can see my baby once they're born?
    - Can you confirm my baby won't leave the operating room unless there is an issue?
    - Will you close my incision with stitches or staples?
- Am I able to have a trial of labor after cesarean (TOLAC) if I want that?

- Do you use forceps or vacuum, or both? What is your rate of using these?
- If my baby is breech, is an external cephalic version and/or vaginal breech birth something you offer?
- What's your philosophy on cervical exams and how often they're done?
- How do you feel about birth plans/preferences?
- If I want to do the following, are you supportive of:
    - Intermittent monitoring if I am low-risk?
    - Laboring, pushing, or birthing in positions that feel best for me, including being upright or off my back?
- Is delayed cord clamping and immediate skin-to-skin standard in your practice and that of your partners?
- If I want my tubes tied or have an IUD or arm implant birth control placed after I give birth, would you be able to do that?

You definitely want to review the questions above about your hospital, but here are some additional tips to help you find the right provider for you:

1. **Review insurance and access.** Does your insurance cover the practice you plan to go to? How easy is it to make an appointment? Is there an online portal to schedule or get in contact for non-urgent needs? Is parking a breeze or a nightmare?

2. **Decide on an OB-GYN or midwife.** I cover the difference on page 9, "Who can help me deliver my baby?" Ask your potential practice if OB-GYNs and midwives work together in that practice, and if so, whether you might expect to see both, including in the hospital, where midwives might be the ones who manage all low-risk patients.

3. **Ask around.** Often your friends can be a wealth of information on who they love (or don't) when it comes to their OB-GYN or mid-

wife. Ask why they feel the way they do. (But only ask people whose opinion you trust!)

4. **No one to ask? Call Labor and Delivery.** This is my favorite insider hack. The labor and delivery nurses see us in all situations, and they know who they'd pick . . . and who they wouldn't. Call and ask for recommendations!

5. **Tread carefully when it comes to Google reviews.** Online reviews are interesting in that they don't always represent the entire picture. Some doctors also have their reviews overrun by folks who might not agree on their views with abortion, for example. You have to take reviews—positive or negative—with a huge grain of salt.

6. **What about males?** If you know a male provider is not right for you, you need to do your best not to go to a practice that employs any men. This is because one of them may be who you see in a pinch, either in the office, if they are on call at the hospital, or in an emergency. I say this having been trained by and working with some amazing male OB-GYNs who I would trust at my own births—so I don't want you to read anything into this other than that I know for some people this choice is important.

7. **Think about race.** I cover this on page 29, "Does the race of my doctor matter?"

8. **Ask the questions.** In addition to the questions about Labor and Delivery above, head to the checklist on page 307 to ask some (or all—that's up to you) questions about how *this* OB-GYN or midwife practices.

9. **And then trust your gut.** Not every personality is the right one for you, and that's OK! You need to see what the vibe is and decide whether you feel this person is someone you can trust with your pregnancy, your baby, and your vagina! If it doesn't feel like a match made in heaven, it's totally OK to switch.

I'M GOING THE HOMEBIRTH/BIRTH CENTER ROUTE—WHAT NOW?

You've reviewed page 4 ("Where can I have my baby?") and now you've settled on a community birth, either at home or in a birth center. You might expect this to be the part where I try to scare you out of this choice and tell you if you give birth at home your baby could die and why would you do this and I can't believe you would even consider it and . . . Yeah, we're not going for that vibe here.

Trust me, when I was in residency and during my first few years in practice, I viewed birth outside of the hospital as the place where safe birth goes to die. Why? Because my perception was skewed as a result of seeing the worst transfers coming into my high-risk academic medical center, and because when you're new in your career you tend to be really concrete and cautious.

I now see more clearly why people choose it—and the secret is that most times, it will go just fine.

However, I also want to emphasize that the best way to do this safely is to set yourself up for success.

Here's my list of questions to ask your homebirth/birth center provider:

- What's the hospital you recommend if I need to be transferred in labor? How close is it? What kind of relationship do you have with the medical team there? How have your patients felt treated by them? Will they allow you to come with me and stay as a support person?
- What supplies and resources do you have here if we need them (i.e., medications for pain or bleeding, resuscitative equipment for baby)?
- How many births have you attended? What is your licensing? Do you have references for patients I can contact to discuss their

experience here? Can I see your statistics on transfers and complications?
- Who is here to help you during my labor and birth? And who covers you if you're with another patient? Where do I go if the center here is full?
- Are you able to give me antibiotics if I have group B strep? Rhogam if needed? Baby medications like vitamin K, eye ointment, and newborn vaccines?
- What criteria do you use to make sure I am safe to birth here?

Additionally, check the following (links can be found in the back of the book):

- Check with your state's medical board to see what is allowed in your state (i.e., can those midwives prescribe or carry lifesaving medications, etc.).
- Verify your midwife's credentials at the American Midwifery Certification Board.

> Curious about reasons you may need to transfer to a hospital and what to know if you do? Head to page 178, "I planned a homebirth and have to transfer in; what should I know?"

Those questions are all straightforward and should not ruffle any feathers. If they do, it might be a clue that you may want to consider a different midwife or birth location. The good news is that many providers have heard these questions before, will be happy to answer them for you, and will appreciate that you are so curious and dedicated to having the safest community birth that you can.

This is my list for you to optimize your own pregnancy for a successful birth at home or in a birth center:

1. **Have the healthiest pregnancy you can.** Exercise and eat well, because we know doing both increases your chances of a successful vaginal delivery.

2. **Don't skip prenatal tests like your gestational diabetes test, testing for anemia (low blood count), or recommended ultrasounds.** It's important to make sure all is well and we're not missing situations where a community birth might put you or your baby at more risk (such as having undiagnosed, uncontrolled gestational diabetes).

3. **Take all the birth prep classes.** Unmedicated labor is no joke, but preparation can get you ready for it and ease some of the unknown. If possible, have a partner or birth support person attend too. Knowing is half the battle.

4. **Really go through those questions on pages 20 and 21.** If something doesn't feel right, it's OK to change course and choose a different provider or location.

5. **Be prepared mentally for a change in plans.** Know that if you end up needing a hospital transfer, even if it's "just" for an epidural, it's OK to feel sad or disappointed. Practice these scenarios in your head, and also spend time during your prenatal care discussing what a transfer looks like so that you are prepared. Trying to keep a flexible, open mind is key. For more on this, see page 178, "I planned a homebirth and have to transfer in; what should I know?"

6. **Mock up a hospital birth plan/preference list in case you do end up needing to transfer.** This can help you feel in control in case your situation changes unexpectedly.

7. **Ask all the questions.** There often is no one way to do things, and one of the benefits of community midwifery care is more time and openness to adapt care to your individual wants and needs. Build a team you trust!

If you've got questions about routine baby medications after birth, head to page 223, "Can you explain why my baby gets shots and eye ointment when they're born?"

SHOULD I HAVE A WATERBIRTH?

A waterbirth is what it sounds like: having your baby in water, usually in an inflatable pool made for this purpose or in a standard tub. This is *not* the same as laboring in the water and then coming out to have your baby "on land"; rather, when I refer to waterbirth in this section, I mean actually birthing your baby in said water. If you want to read more about laboring in water, head to page 116, "What is the best position to labor in?"

I will tell you that most OB-GYNs—me included—have never cared for a patient who gave birth in a tub. Here's why:

1. Patients who usually want this have traditionally chosen midwives, not us.
2. Our governing organizations (like the American College of Obstetricians and Gynecologists and the American Academy of Pediatrics) have said that while they support laboring in water, babies should be born on land. They say we don't have enough studies to show it's safe, so this means that most hospitals we work in don't offer it.

But are those safety concerns real? Hmm . . .

Speaking as someone who's been trained in a system that scared me off waterbirth, I acknowledge my biases. However, as better and more data emerges, we need to be willing to adapt our opinion. And we also need to know why our patients may want something and to be able to give them accurate information so they can make an informed choice.

With that said: Why might someone want a waterbirth, and are there any risks or benefits? Let's see . . .

Potential benefits	**Has this been shown in studies?**	**Dr. Jen's notes**
Less pain	Yes	This was defined as lower pain medication use in labor.
More satisfied with the birth process	Yes	This isn't something to overlook, as we know birth can be traumatizing.
Shorter time spent pushing	Unclear	
Less tearing	Unclear	
Fewer episiotomies	Yes	Makes sense—hard to cut what you can't see.
Feels more gentle and natural	I don't think we need studies to look at this	

Potential risks	**Has this been shown in studies?**	**Dr. Jen's notes**
Increased infection in mom	No	
Increased risk of postpartum hemorrhage	No	The risk might actually be *lower* in the water.
Increased infection in baby	Yes . . . and no	Some cases have been reported from waterborne bacteria, but poor sanitary conditions were the likely cause. Other studies showed 36% *fewer* infections in these babies.

Potential risks	Has this been shown in studies?	Dr. Jen's notes
Water aspiration in baby (drowning from breathing underwater)	No	A recent analysis actually showed a 40% *decrease* in the risk of aspiration and NICU admission.
Hypothermia in baby	No	The water temperature should be closely monitored to keep it in a safe range.
The umbilical cord snaps off (cord avulsion)	Yes; the risk is about 1 in 290 waterbirths vs. 1 in 1,300 land births	This seems like a pretty easy thing to avoid by being careful.

So based on our most recent evidence synthesized in 2024—which is ever-evolving—**waterbirth is likely very safe for the low-risk pregnant person.** Other than an increased risk of cord avulsion (which is still uncommon), the benefits might just outweigh the risks.

The most important thing to do if you want a waterbirth is to have a midwife or OB-GYN who is on board with the plan and birthing in a hospital where you know it's offered. This is a great thing to figure out early on in your pregnancy.

"WILL MY BABY BREATHE UNDERWATER?"

Most babies don't breathe when they're swimming in water, whether that's amniotic fluid or at the time of a waterbirth. This is because breathing is usually suppressed because of hormones and the dive reflex. A distressed baby may try to breathe, though, and this is why monitoring for that is important to make a waterbirth safer.

WILL MY INSURANCE FOR MY OB-GYN COVER EVERYTHING . . . LIKE MY EPIDURAL?

You have no idea how annoyed I am that this is something we have to worry about in the United States . . . and yet we do. The answer is a big *no*—which is why I am addressing it.

Yes, it is certainly possible that your health insurance covers your prenatal care, your OB-GYN's delivery fees, and all the costs associated with your hospital stay. But you *cannot* assume that. For example, some plans may cover it all, while others might only partially cover ultrasounds, genetic screening, and more.

Another thing to know is that your insurance may not cover everyone you see in the hospital (yes, really). For example, the anesthesiologist who places your epidural or the urologist who might consult during your C-section may actually be out-of-network for you.

Scary, right? Because how many of us are stopping in the midst of painful contractions to ask the anesthesia team if they're in network with our health plan? (I can tell you I certainly didn't!) Or mid-operation say, "Wait! Please check if you're in network before you scrub in!" Only in America . . .

Frustration aside, you *can* prepare by closely examining your health insurance benefits. To know if your (possible) epidural might be covered, you can ask your OB-GYN what anesthesia group works on Labor and Delivery, then call them and ask if they are in-network in your plan, or if you need a prior authorization (which of course you want to do well *before* you go into labor). You can also ask for a written good-faith estimate, which allows you to know what your out-of-pocket cost might be.

Keep in mind that if more than one anesthesia practice covers Labor and Delivery and an out-of-network one happens to be on staff the day you need your epidural, it's likely you'll get a bill that's higher than one from a practice that's in-network. You can't really control which day you go into labor, so isn't that just an amazing little tidbit? You can often fight this with your insurance company afterward, but it usually isn't straightforward or easy, and they may not refund you the full cost.

I'm not sharing this to scare or depress you; I just want you to be informed ahead of time, so you aren't hit with shock if you get an unexpected bill.

There's enough to worry about when you're pregnant, and what your insurance pays or doesn't shouldn't be one of them. If I could wave a magic wand and make this go away, trust me, I would. Until then, know your doctors hate this part of medicine and we will keep fighting to make it better for you.

DOES THE RELIGIOUS AFFILIATION OF MY HOSPITAL MATTER?

It sure can.

This mainly applies when we're talking about Catholic hospitals, where more than 500,000 babies are born every year. This accounts for 16 percent of all hospital births nationwide—but in the state of Washington, that number is actually 50 percent. So it depends where you live.

Catholic hospitals are bound by a set of rules called the "Ethical and Religious Directives for Catholic Care Services." The rules are authored by Catholic bishops, whose nonmedical writings dictate how healthcare is provided.

In it, they write:

- "Abortion . . . is never permitted."
- "Catholic health institutions may not promote or condone contraceptive practices but should provide, for married couples and the medical staff who counsel them, instruction . . . about the Church's teaching on . . . natural family planning."

- "Direct sterilization of either men or women, whether permanent or temporary, is not permitted in a Catholic health care institution."

These directives mean that your OB-GYN may not be able to give you the healthcare or treatment you need, such as an abortion if your bag of water breaks before your baby can live outside the uterus and if they still have a heartbeat. This can lead to needing to be transferred to a different hospital with doctors you don't know and potentially getting sick or dying from a delay in care.

It can also mean that if you're done having kids and request that a tubal ligation be done at the time of your C-section, your doctor's hands may be tied, and she won't be allowed to do it. Or if you want an IUD or Nexplanon (implantable birth control that goes in your arm) placed prior to your discharge, that may not be permissible.

You might be thinking, "Well, if you want those things, then don't choose a Catholic hospital!" If that choice is available to you, I completely agree. However, this freedom to choose isn't always possible, such as:

- When your employer offers only one type of health insurance, and it's a Catholic hospital's plan.
- If an ambulance takes you to a Catholic hospital in an emergency, you don't really have a say.
- If the only hospital that's in reasonable driving distance is a Catholic one.
- The hospital website doesn't disclose that they are Catholic. (21 percent of Catholic hospital websites do not!)

The reality is that with four of the ten largest hospital chains in the country being Catholic hospitals, in some states only a Catholic hospital may be accessible to you.

In a post-*Roe* world, access to care matters now more than ever, which is why I am including this section in my book. I *do* want to point out that some Catholic hospitals are less restrictive than others when it comes to interpreting the directives: Some will offer abortion if it is medically necessary (though it needs to be cleared by an ethics committee—something that I, as a trained medical professional, find highly insulting), and some may offer contraception and tubal ligations.

My take-home message: If you're planning to birth at a Catholic hospital, it's worth clarifying what is—and isn't—available to you long before you show up in labor.

DOES THE RACE OF MY DOCTOR MATTER?

It can, and in the United States, where racism plays a major role in obstetric and neonatal outcomes, it is worth considering if you are a nonwhite person.

Black women are . . .

- Three to four times more likely to die from pregnancy-associated causes than white women (nine times higher in New York City)
- Twice as likely to have a baby born preterm
- Twice as likely to have their concerns ignored
- Sixty percent more likely to be diagnosed with preeclampsia
- Twenty-two percent more likely to report obstetric violence (more on this on page 272—"I think I had a traumatic birth and I don't know where to go for help")

Indigenous women are . . .

- Twice as likely to die from pregnancy-associated causes than white women

Black babies are . . .

- Half as likely to die by their first birthday when cared for by Black doctors

It's important to note that these numbers can't be written off as a result of worse access to care or lower education levels. Studies have shown us this time and time again.

I also want to highlight that **race itself is not the risk factor**. Yes, there is evidence of what's known as the weathering theory, whereby stressors can play a role in your genetics and thus can be passed down in families, but the vast majority of these worse outcomes for nonwhite birthing people is due to *racism* as the risk factor—not race.

This plays out as Black women not being treated for pain as often as their white counterparts. Or increased rates of Black babies being placed in the foster care system—which, when you know this, might lead you to be fearful about calling your doctor if you have a concern. It's the fact that Black women are more often criminalized for their miscarriages.

This is not a feel-good section, but it doesn't mean you can't *do* something to counteract these statistics. One way is to get your care with someone who has the same racial background and lived experience as you. Studies show us patients get better care and speak up more often in these scenarios.

The unfortunate reality is that finding a doctor who matches your racial or ethnic background might be challenging depending on where you live, as these numbers from 2022 show us:

Race	Percentage of doctors in the United States
White	56.5%
Asian	18.8%
Hispanic/Latinx	6.3%
Black	5.2%
Multiracial	1.3%
American Indian/Alaska Native	0.3%
Native Hawaiian/Pacific Islander	0.1%
Other	1.1%
Unknown	10.4%

Another option—and an important one if you can't find a doctor or midwife who looks like you—is to have a doula who shares your race or ethnicity. I cover doulas much more in the next section, so check that out.

Lastly, there is no question that we have work to do in our field. You shouldn't have to carry this burden. Or the burden of knowing you might have to speak up more to be heard (see page 138, "I don't feel I'm being listened to. What are my options?"). It's OK to be angry that this is birth in America and also be armed with some actionable ways to take control and get the birth you want and deserve.

DO I NEED A DOULA?

Doulas can be a fantastic addition to your birth team! But in truth, not everybody wants or needs one. Some folks feel that having someone in the room who isn't their partner is invasive, and others may feel it is unnecessary because they feel the support of their partner (or other family members or friends) is enough. So, the choice to have a doula is entirely up to you!

I do want to clarify up front that doulas are *not* the same as midwives and do not manage labor or have the same medical training. But they can be a great complement to a midwife or doctor.

Doulas are trained professionals who provide support before, during, and after birth with the goal of helping you have an informed and empowered birth. Their support can be both physical (working with you in labor to help alleviate pain and find positions to help your labor progress) and emotional (such as reassuring you and cheering you on when you feel like you can't go on another minute). Doulas can attend your prenatal visits with you and can also provide postpartum support in your home.

A huge part of what doulas do is education, especially since they often spend so much more time with you—in pregnancy while you prepare, and again postpartum—than you usually get at your OB-GYN or midwife visits. They can help demystify birth and prep you on what to expect, as well as help you advocate for what you need. And since they're seeing you in your own home, without the time constraints of a clinic appointment, they can often go deeper in explanations while also helping you formulate questions for your medical team.

One of my favorite roles that doulas perform is as your advocate. They can:

- Ask the questions you may have forgotten or are too distracted to ask
- Help communicate your birth preferences to your team
- Interpret to you what may have sounded like complicated medical jargon
- Be a great voice for someone who may feel they can't ask certain questions out of fear of being labeled "difficult" (it's ridiculous that some people are made to feel this way; trust me, it's not OK)

Does this sound like a bunch of earthy natural crunchy stuff? Well, it's not! **There is data to show that having a trained doula as part of your birth team can lead to a shorter labor, lower C-section and vacuum/forceps rates, less need for pain medication, and higher birth satisfaction.** In my role as an OB-GYN, if I had a medicine that did all that, I'd prescribe it to every pregnant person I ever came into contact with!

One last note on doulas: The kinds of doulas who showed those amazing results above had training and experience. That is, there's a huge difference between a certified doula and someone who calls herself a doula because she's had a baby before. If you are curious on how to find a trained doula, the Doula Association of North America (DONA) is a great place to start (see page 297). You can also ask your obstetric provider if your hospital provides doulas (some do, free of charge) or if they have ones in particular that they recommend.

CAN I JUST REQUEST A C-SECTION?

Yes, you can . . . but: It doesn't mean your OB-GYN is going to be OK or excited about doing it. Let's talk about why.

C-sections, while common (and lifesaving when used appropriately), are a major abdominal surgery. If you deliver by C-section, you are more likely to:

- Lose more blood
- Get an infection
- Develop blood clots
- Need an emergency hysterectomy (removal of the uterus)
- Stay in the hospital longer
- Have a longer and harder recovery

Babies born via C-section also have some unique risks. They are more likely to need help breathing when they're first born (because they don't get all the amniotic fluid squeezed out of their lungs like babies who make their way down the birth canal do). This may mean they need help from a breathing mask, or even be admitted to the NICU for a short while.

A C-section also makes your next deliveries a bit higher-risk, as it increases your risk in subsequent pregnancies of:

- Uterine rupture (where the prior scar opens—an absolute emergency, though rare at about 0.5 to 1 percent)
- Placenta previa (where the placenta covers the cervix and can bleed, sometimes leading to an early emergent delivery)
- Placenta accreta (where the placenta abnormally attaches to the wall of the uterus; a hysterectomy at time of delivery is often the treatment)

These risks after having one C-section are small but definitely go up substantially the more C-sections you have. For example, if you've had two C-sections and have a placenta previa in your third pregnancy, there is a 40 percent chance you'll also have a placenta accreta and need a cesarean hysterectomy, which is a potentially life-threatening surgery. That's pretty significant!

It's not fair if I don't discuss the benefits of a scheduled C-section, though, so we must cover that too. A planned C-section means:

- Your birth can be scheduled, whereas labor often can't.
- There's no guarantee that if you labor you won't end up with a C-section anyway.
- You avoid pushing, potential vaginal tearing, and complications like shoulder dystocia.
- You might be able to avoid pelvic organ prolapse and urinary leakage later in life, since we know that vaginal delivery changes your pelvic floor and increases your risk of these complications.

So, should you ask for a scheduled C-section? It's up to you, but I'd want you to think about *why* you're wanting to go this route. Are you scared of the pain of labor? If so, we can talk about that (see page 107 for more). Does the idea of labor totally freak you out? That's OK—you aren't alone, and sometimes talking with a therapist can help you address this. How many kids do you want to have? Because if it's three, four, or more, a C-section can really set you up for some high-risk births in the future.

It's important you communicate why you're thinking of a C-section and discuss this sooner rather than later with your obstetric provider, so that you can have a plan and really think through all your options.

IF I'VE HAD A C-SECTION BEFORE, SHOULD I HAVE ONE AGAIN?

You have two choices if you've had a prior C-section: to have a repeat C-section, or to have a trial of labor after cesarean (TOLAC) with the goal of having a vaginal birth after cesarean (VBAC). (We love our abbreviations in obstetrics.)

Before I jump into the risks and benefits of each choice, I want you to know the following:

1. **Not all hospitals routinely offer TOLACs.** This is because in order to offer one in the safest way, the ability to perform an emergency C-section must be available, and not all hospitals have an OB-GYN and/or anesthesiologist present in the hospital 24/7.
2. **Despite that, you can't be forced into a C-section.** Even the American College of Obstetricians and Gynecologists says that coercion is unacceptable, no one can be forced into a surgery, and choosing to have a TOLAC in a hospital without the above resources should be "carefully considered" between doctor and patient—not refused

outright. This is obviously something to discuss long before you're in labor, so that an informed conversation can be had.

3. **Not all C-sections are the same.** Whether or not your doctor recommends a TOLAC will depend on the type of C-section you previously had. If you've had the kind called a classical C-section (where the incision on the uterus is vertical), they will not recommend any future laboring or vaginal births because of the increased risk of uterine rupture with these types of prior incisions. It's also important to know that certain types of uterine surgery also drastically increase this risk, so your doctor will also review your history with you. (The kind of incision on your belly does not tell us what kind of incision you had on your uterus.)

4. **How many C-sections you've had matters.** Current guidelines tell us it is safe to try for a TOLAC after one or two prior C-sections. If you've had more than this, you likely won't find an OB-GYN who feels comfortable with a TOLAC because of an increased risk of uterine rupture.

5. **Attempting a TOLAC outside of a hospital is not recommended.** For the reasons you'll see below, the hospital is seen by leading medical organizations as the safest place to undergo a TOLAC. However, I know that some people still may choose to birth at home or in a birth center. The midwives who care for these patients have a responsibility to inform their patients of the risks and alternatives available and, if patients still choose to not birth in a hospital, to ensure emergency transfer is available insofar as possible.

As I've been hinting at, the main concern with a TOLAC is the risk of **uterine rupture.** This is when the uterus opens up along the prior C-section scar. It can result in a rupture (full-thickness separation, where the baby can actually come out of the uterus) or a dehiscence (where the uterine muscle is thin and we can often see through it, but it's not fully separated). This is a life-threatening emergency for both you and your baby, and the treatment is an emergency C-section (along with a hysterectomy if bleeding cannot be controlled).

This sounds scary, but thankfully it's rare, complicating 0.5 percent of all TOLACs—that is, fewer than 1 in 100. With an induction of labor that number is a bit higher but still remains low, at approximately 1 in 100. In labor, we purposely avoid using misoprostol and dinoprostone (drugs used for cervical ripening), which are known to increase this risk further; more about them on page 80, "How does an induction work?" We also continuously monitor your fetus in labor when you're having a TOLAC, as one of the first signs of uterine rupture can be a dramatic drop in your baby's heart rate.

So, let's talk about the risks and benefits of both of your options:

	Benefits	**Risks**
Scheduled repeat C-section	• You know when your baby is arriving (probably). • You don't have to go through labor. • You avoid the chance of trying for a TOLAC only to end up with a C-section anyway.	• Major abdominal surgery with higher complication risks compared to a vaginal birth; see the section above for more. • Makes your future pregnancies higher-risk. • You may go into labor before your scheduled C-section, so you can't guarantee your delivery date.
Undergoing a trial of labor after cesarean (TOLAC)	• If you have a successful TOLAC, you have all the benefits of a vaginal birth, such as a quicker recovery and lower risk of complications as compared to a C-section. • Can feel empowering for someone who wanted to achieve a vaginal birth and didn't in their prior pregnancy. • Avoiding more C-sections if you're planning a large family can decrease your risk in future pregnancies and births.	• You may labor but still end up with a C-section (and these are the births with the highest risks to you and baby). • Uterine rupture could occur.

If you're unsure of what path to choose, knowing what your estimated rate of success at having a vaginal birth would be can help inform you. Factors that play into this can include the reason for your prior C-section (was it because your baby was breech or because your baby didn't fit?), if you've had vaginal births before, if you have gestational diabetes this time around, and more.

While imperfect, calculators do exist that can help us guide this discussion with you (you can find them in the Resources section on page 297). However, it's important to note you don't have to achieve a certain score on a test like this in order to be "allowed" to try for a VBAC—it's just meant to help inform your decision. It's also OK to not use these calculators if you feel like you want a TOLAC regardless and a lower score will stress you out.

Whether or not to have a TOLAC or repeat C-section is a personal choice, and my goal is that you feel informed to have these conversations with your provider. If you feel like you're being met with resistance, I strongly encourage you to share the references for this section and ask your doctor to read through them thoroughly to understand where you're coming from. I say this because, sadly, a lot of misinformation and scare tactics still exist around vaginal birth after cesarean, and you deserve to have an evidence-based team on your side.

WHO SHOULD I HAVE WITH ME IN THE ROOM ON THE BIG DAY?

This is a personal decision, but before you even start thinking about who you want to invite to the birthday party, you need to know if your hospital has any rules. That is, are you allowed only two support people, or is the sky the limit? This is a great thing to ask when considering where you might want to have your baby—see page 14, "I've chosen a hospital—what should I ask about?"

That said, here's what I recommend when deciding who will be at your labor and birth:

1. **Only have people who can see and hear everything.** Are you OK with them seeing you naked, peeing, pooping, and throwing up? While these might not all happen (and we try to have support folks step out during sensitive moments), sometimes we don't have time to ensure Grandpa won't see your vulva in an emergency.

2. **Don't invite people who will make it all about them.** I can't tell you the number of times an aunt or mom has turned the big moment into theirs, and it got real awkward for everyone involved. How do you know who will do this? If you automatically thought of someone when reading this, that might be a sign . . .

3. **Do you want a party or an intimate moment?** There's no right or wrong answer here. Be true to what you and your partner want, not what others are pressuring you to do.

4. **Consider a doula** (see page 31 for more on this), knowing that doulas can be amazing but also aren't for everyone. Whatever feels right to you is your right answer.

5. **When do you want people there?** Do you want some visitors to stop by during labor but step out for the actual birth? Or do you want them there for the whole thing? Be sure to communicate your preferences ahead of time so that feelings don't get hurt and you don't have to deal with it as your baby is crowning.

6. **Think about your rest.** Sometimes labor takes a while (especially inductions, which can take days). Do you want people there the whole time? Are they interfering with your sleep or rest? Are they making you feel like a watched pot that never boils?

7. **Siblings and younger family members.** Having kids present (like older siblings of the baby you're birthing) is something you should think through. I have been at some beautiful births where a big

sister gets to welcome her baby brother to the world, and it had everyone in tears. I've also had a pregnant person who needed an emergency C-section and the partner had no one else available to care for the sibling, so the partner had to stay out of the OR and miss the birth. My advice is to consider each child's age and personality (will they be scared if they see you in pain?) and make sure there is another adult whose sole responsibility is that kiddo if an emergency arises, for both their comfort and their safety. And of course, check to see if there's an age limit for visitors at your hospital.

I want you to know that whatever you decide, **you get to change your mind as many times as you want**—this is *your* experience, not any visitors' or wannabe visitors'. Whatever you need, let your nurses and providers know. We are more than happy to speak up on your behalf and go to bat for you.

WHEN SHOULD I PICK A PEDIATRICIAN?

Before conception.

Just kidding—it's not like daycare! But ideally, having your pediatrician (or family practice doctor) selected before your baby arrives is recommended so that you won't be scrambling on the day you're getting discharged from the hospital.

Many pediatricians offer no-charge "meet and greet" appointments for pregnant folks, when you can see the office, chat with the doctor, and ultimately see if they are a good fit for your family. This can be done anytime during your pregnancy, but most people tend to do them in the second or third trimester.

Because I happen to be married to a pediatrician who is much more experienced in this than I am, here's the list of questions Dr. Doug recommends when picking out your baby's doctor:

Head to page 311 for a checklist you can use at a pediatrician meet-and-greet visit.

QUESTIONS FOR THE PEDIATRICIAN-TO-BE:

1. **How accessible are you and how easy is it to make appointments?** Oftentimes, you can find this information on the practice's website, but it's worth asking the following:

   - Can I schedule an appointment for an acute issue on the same day?
   - Is the clinic open on weekends?
   - What happens if I have a question in the middle of the night?
   - Who answers the phone during business hours when I have a clinical question?
   - Do you have an online portal where I can send in questions?
   - Do you offer telehealth visits?
   - How many days a week do you see patients?
   - If I'm not seeing you, who fills in?

2. **Will I see you in the hospital?** Some pediatricians come in to meet their newest patients and do newborn rounds, while others won't see you until you come in to the office. In the latter case, when your baby is born, a hospital-employed pediatrician will instead see your baby and make sure all the important information gets sent to your eventual pediatrician.

3. **What support can I expect here?** A good pediatric practice functions as a medical home for your child. You can ask questions like:

   - Do you have a lactation consultant, a social worker, therapists, or behavioral specialists available?
   - If I need referrals elsewhere, do you have someone who coordinates this and makes it easy?

4. **What is your communication style?** A good pediatrician will be able to tailor his or her recommendations to your needs, but at the end of the day we all have our unique personalities. Do you think you're someone who wants to know a by-the-minute sleep schedule and exactly how many ounces of sweet potato puree your baby should be eating at six months, or does that level of detail stress you out and you prefer a more laid-back approach? It's kind of like dating, where you want to find the right personality match, and it's OK to swipe left on a doctor who doesn't seem to get your style.

5. **What's the best part of your job?** Does this seem like a strange thing to ask when trying to pick a doctor? I don't think so, and it's because this question helps you understand their philosophy and how you can expect them to show up for your child. My husband went into pediatrics for three reasons: He loves the breadth of knowledge he must know in primary care, he loves getting to know kids and families and watching them grow up, and it's really fun for him to play with kids and connect with teens all day. Most pediatricians will have a variation of this answer. Look for passion and a sense of meaning in caring for your kids.

6. **Can you help with my medically complex child?** If you know your little one is going to need some extra care because of a prenatal diagnosis, this can be important to address. Has the doctor taken care of kids with this issue before? Do you get the sense they know the pediatric subspecialists you'll need to see, and can help with referrals and care coordination? Or do they seem to have a deer-in-the-headlights look when you ask?

WHAT IF I HAVE CONCERNS ABOUT VACCINES?

Some practices will not care for kids unless they are fully vaccinated. If you plan to not vaccinate your child or pursue a non-evidence-based vaccine schedule, you should clarify this prenatally so that you aren't left without a doctor for your baby unexpectedly once they arrive. I do want to say here that both my husband and I fully believe that vaccinating on schedule is safe and can be lifesaving. Vaccines have prevented millions of deaths and are one of the best public health interventions we have. And yes, our kids are fully vaccinated, including flu shots and COVID boosters! He also believes that children who are not fully vaccinated deserve access to healthcare, and thus works hard to partner with families to make sure they feel heard, can communicate their concerns, and make a decision that is based on science, data, and trust—not on misinformation.

Once you've had the meet-and-greet visit, here are some questions for you:

1. **What was the vibe?** Your baby will have at least eight visits with this doc before they turn one year old, so did you feel comfortable with them? Can you be yourself? Does this pediatrician seem to listen to you? Seem to care about who you are? Asks about your goals and worries with having a baby? Has a sense of humor? Basically, what's your gut after meeting the pediatrician?
2. **How did the office feel?** First impressions matter. You will be spending *a lot* of time in this office. Was parking a nightmare? Does the office feel comfortable and welcoming? Is check-in smooth? Are the nurses and medical assistants kind? Even if you have the best doctor in the world, if scheduling appointments is hard and the clinic isn't convenient, maybe this isn't the place for you.
3. **A word on Google reviews.** These can be . . . interesting. You can certainly scroll through them, but note that these don't always reflect the views of the majority of patients.

Do you have to do all this work before you give birth? Absolutely not. You're busy growing a human, and if this falls off the list, don't worry about it. You can ask your obstetric provider or your friends who they recommend. Often one of the best resources are the hospital nurses. They interact with many pediatricians and can tell you who their faves are.

And remember, you can always switch if you don't click with the person or practice once your baby arrives.

SHOULD I MAKE A BIRTH PLAN . . . OR DOES EVERY OB-GYN HATE THEM?

Birth plans *definitely* have a reputation in the obstetric community, and unfortunately, it's usually not a good one. The story is often about the twelve-page laminated birth plan that includes things like "Don't ever ask me if I want an epidural, and even if I am begging for one you must ask my husband's permission. And don't make direct eye contact. And if I need a C-section it must only be done by candlelight so it feels calm. And . . ." Yeah. You see where I'm going.

The reality is that when we make fun of birth plans, we lose focus on why they are made—which is because birth *has* been overmedicalized. People feel a lack of safety or control. They don't feel heard. And if they're Black or brown, they are worried they may not survive birth.

It's serious stuff. It's not a joke.

So, let's come at this from a different angle: Birth plans mean our patients have thought about their labor, are informed, and want to be heard. How amazing! Let's encourage that.

For the pregnant person reading this, I would then say yes—let's see what is important to you! I'd also recommend reframing your birth plan as your *birth preferences*, knowing that sometimes even the best plan requires some flexibility.

I also cannot stress enough that **you should review this with your OB-GYN or midwife during your pregnancy,** to ensure that the things you are wanting and hoping for are available and noted.

Another reason to review your birth plan at your prenatal visits is to see if your provider passes the vibe check. If your doctor balks at the existence of your birth plan at your twenty-eight-week checkup, you've got more than enough time to find a new provider before your due date.

Now on to what you should actually include if you choose to have a birth plan (and not having one is just fine, too). I've seen *a lot* of birth plans/preferences, and it often surprises me how so many templates are out of date. There's a lot of requests for us to not do things that haven't been done in a long time, and this sometimes makes it hard to focus in on what is truly important to someone. There's no need to request not having an enema, shave, or routine episiotomy—these are old practices that (thankfully) are no longer the standard, so you can leave these off yours. But if you're worried enough, or have heard in the community that, say, episiotomy rates are really high (more on page 205), then by all means include it.

You can Google a birth plan and find limitless options, but some are better than others. Here's what I recommend if you want to make one:

1. **Keep it short and sweet.** This makes it much more likely to be read from start to finish.

2. **Make it accessible.** Bring a copy to a prenatal appointment and ask that it be scanned into your chart. You should also bring a few copies to the hospital so that there's one for your nurse, one for your OB-GYN or midwife, and extras in case there are shift changes or they get lost in the shuffle.

3. **Include what matters to *you*.** You don't need to check all the boxes or request things that aren't a priority. Including what you really want or need ensures it's prioritized.

4. **Talk it up.** Proactively ask to review it with your hospital team, including after every shift change so that new team members are in the loop. This can be a great job for your partner to do with every new team member who comes into the room.

5. **If you've had a traumatic birth before, tell us.** I cover how to prevent repeated birth trauma on page 176, "I had a traumatic birth before and I want to know how to have a better experience this time," and one of the best things you can do is tell us what happened before and what you need this time.

6. **Consider using my birth preference template** (page 301). Like I said, lots of options exist, and this is just one more—but I think a birth plan template written by an OB-GYN who has seen a lot and wants you to have the birth you deserve is one you should consider!

IS IT TIME?

WHEN THE OB-GYN GETS SENT HOME FROM TRIAGE

I was pregnant with my second baby and two days shy of my due date. Having painful contractions, I went to see my OB-GYN in clinic to see if it was time. I found out I was 4 centimeters dilated, which sounds great—but I knew, since it wasn't my first, that this wasn't a guarantee I was actually in labor.

I headed to triage afterward with my husband to see if there was any more cervical change. We already had our sibling doula at home with our son, and he was excited to hear he might wake up with a baby brother to meet. Unfortunately, my cervix was not any more dilated when we got to triage, so we went for a walk for an hour or two. I almost threw up in a garbage can at one point because I was so uncomfortable. This had to be it!

And then . . . the contractions stopped.

I knew it meant now was not actually the day I'd be staying and having a baby. I was so bummed out. How was I going to go home, be potentially uncomfortable, and have to arrange the childcare situation *again* when it actually was time? And deal with a very disappointed kiddo at home?

Yet I went home, still very pregnant, knowing it was the right thing to do but also feeling very much like a failure. Of all people, an OB-GYN couldn't figure out when she was in labor? And would I be pregnant for *weeks* longer? I was an emotional wreck.

A few days later, it was in fact time, and everything turned out just fine. But I share this to say: If you feel like your body is confusing you or letting you down, you are not alone. Even the board-certified doctor can't predict it all, so I beg you to go easy on yourself if you too get sent home from triage.

HOW DO I KNOW WHEN TO GO TO THE HOSPITAL?

Let me start by saying that it's perfectly OK to go to the hospital thinking you are in labor only to get sent home. You didn't get it wrong. You're not the only person this has happened to. Sometimes it's hard to know, and we would 100 percent rather you come in and get checked out than sit home and worry.

With that out of the way, here are the reasons you should *absolutely* come to Labor and Delivery:

1. Your bag of water has broken.

2. Your contractions are regular (i.e., every five minutes), they're painful, and you can't talk through them.

3. Your baby isn't moving at all, or not as they have been, and you're worried.

4. You're bleeding heavily, or enough to worry you.

That's a pretty short list, right? That's because there are few absolutes in medicine, and in birth especially.

The following are "maybe" reasons. The next step with these is often to call your provider to talk it through and figure out what to do next (I cover how to contact them in the next section):

1. **You're having contractions . . . but not sure if it's "bad enough."** Maybe they're painful but only fifteen minutes apart. Or maybe they're every five minutes, but just light cramps.

2. **You've had spotting.** Spotting can be normal and expected after things like sex or a membrane sweep, so it may not mean you have to come in—but it's worth a call to know.

3. **You think you lost your mucus plug or you're having more mucus discharge.** It's true that having more mucus discharge or what looks like snot (yes, really) can be a sign your cervix is dilating, but it does not guarantee labor is on the way. For most folks at term, we'd tell you this alone is not a reason to come to the hospital. However, if you're preterm or if it's got you worried, you should give us a call, as we may ask you to come in.

4. **You leaked fluid when you sneezed once.** This is probably urine and not your bag of water, but if it's unclear, we may ask you to come in to get checked.

Note: These scenarios are only for term, low-risk pregnancies. If you are less than 37 weeks or have a high-risk pregnancy, you should definitely check in with your provider and follow their recommendations. Also, if something feels off or if you feel like you must be seen, then you always have the right to come in and get evaluated!

WHO CAN I CALL AT 3 A.M. ON A SUNDAY IF I HAVE QUESTIONS?

This might be one of the *first* questions I want you to ask your OB-GYN or midwife when you establish care. Can you hear me through the pages of this book? Be sure to ask this question! And if the answer is "We don't have a number, you just call Labor and Delivery," I am going to put myself out there and say that I don't love that.

Why? Because a practice that cares for pregnant people, whether it is a huge multispecialty group or a tiny clinic with two private-practice OB-GYNs in a rural community, should have a way to be reachable *all the time*. Babies come at 3 A.M., on Sundays, on the Fourth of July, and during snowstorms. And concerns like you've fallen or you're not sure if your water broke don't only happen during office hours.

You deserve to be able to call someone who knows you (or at least knows of you) for advice whenever you need it. (Reality check: Please don't call your doctor's answering service at 2 A.M. for a birth control refill. I do beg you to let that one be a daytime phone call.)

With all of this in mind, your provider should have an on-call number that you can call after hours. Often an answering service will take your message and page (yes, we still use pagers) your doctor or midwife or whoever is on call for them at that moment, who will then call you back. This step is important because it can also keep you out of the hospital if you're able to chat with someone who can review your symptoms and reassure you that it's OK to stay at home—unlike a labor and delivery nurse, who in many states is not legally able to give you advice if you call other than telling you that you can come in to be seen if you're worried.

Important note: If you're having a true emergency, just come on in. Don't worry about looking for that number. But for other scenarios, get this number and make sure you, your partner, and any support folks have it in their phones for when you need it.

I'M GOING OUT OF TOWN AND I'M PREGNANT—WHAT SHOULD I DO JUST IN CASE?

You're trying to fit in that babymoon . . . but what do you need to think about before you travel somewhere amazingly gorgeous and romantic? You know I love a list:

1. **Is abortion accessible where you're going?** If you just whiplashed so fast at reading that, here's why I am including that and putting it at number one. The reality is that complications happen. What if you're in Texas at 18 weeks gestation, your bag of water breaks, you

start to get sick, and the treatment is abortion (whether via surgery to empty the uterus or medical treatment), but the hospital won't allow it because of their abortion ban? Sure, they might eventually do it if you're sick "enough," but do you want to risk getting septic and losing organs? Or having to be sent via medical helicopter to a state that allows this care? Yeah, this question is a drag, but sometimes the reality of being pregnant in America is just that.

2. **Confirm you're safe to travel.** It doesn't hurt to check in with your OB-GYN or midwife before traveling far from home, but this really applies to high-risk pregnancies. Of note, airlines are wildly inconsistent on when they say you can fly until (and honestly, some of those rules seem so random to me). Be sure to check your airline's website to see what they say and if you may need a note confirming your due date so that you don't get turned away at the gate.

3. **Check for any travel advisories.** Remember Zika virus? If not, it's OK (and now I just feel old), but the point is, sometimes there are outbreaks of diseases in certain locations that make traveling there potentially dangerous if you're pregnant. You can find this information by searching for Centers for Disease Control and U.S. Department of State travel advisories, with the caveat that these no longer may be as accurate as they once were.

4. **Have the basics written down somewhere.** Just in case an emergency arises and you're too stressed or unable to communicate the basics, have a few facts written down and kept in your wallet or on your phone so that they can be referenced. Include your name, date of birth, due date, what number pregnancy this is for you, any high-risk issues this pregnancy, if you've had a C-section before, and the name and contact information of your obstetric provider.

5. **Know the closest labor and delivery unit.** Yes, you could Google it quickly if a situation arises, but why not have the hospital name and number ahead of time so you don't have to worry?

VERY IMPORTANT: Not all hospitals have a labor and delivery unit, so confirm this on their website or by calling before just heading in. This can save you precious time and stress.

6. **Consider only traveling somewhere you'd be OK having your baby.** Some pregnancy complications mean being hospitalized until you give birth. This means if you travel to a different state or country at 23 weeks gestation and have an issue, you may be advised to stay there until after your baby arrives. Thankfully, this is rare, but every OB-GYN has managed a patient who has been through this (including myself, more than once). Think through what this could mean for you in terms of healthcare costs, your job, potentially being separated from other children, and being in an environment where you may not know anyone or speak the language.

This list isn't meant to alarm you, but rather just to help you be prepared and clarify for you what level of uncertainty is acceptable for you.

Don't forget to wear sunscreen!

WHAT SHOULD I HAVE IN MY LABOR AND DELIVERY BAG?

I love social media, but some of the TikToks that highlight these excessive hospital bags make me cringe. You are packing to go have a baby, not for a world tour—let's not make this overcomplicated!

If you're a minimalist at heart, here is my list for you:

What you should bring
Your ID
Your insurance card
Baby car seat (before discharge)
A copy of your birth plan/preferences
This book!
What can be nice to have
Stuff to keep you entertained (especially during a labor induction): a book, magazine, your laptop, etc., and all chargers
Stuff to keep you comfy: a playlist, some battery-powered candles, personal toiletries, slippers, a bathrobe or PJs you don't mind throwing out afterward, a white-noise machine or phone app (the hospital can be noisy)
Stuff to keep you full: snacks or drinks you like
Stuff for after: a comfy nursing bra, an outfit for baby, and a maternity outfit for you going home (regular clothes won't fit yet—that's OK!)

You can always bring more with you, but this is meant to be practical and not induce a ton of stress.

Let me say one thing about gifts for your nurses or doctor: We don't need them. We really don't want you to spend your last few weeks of pregnancy worrying about assembling complicated gift bags for us. If you feel you must do something, leave us a good review and send us a baby announcement so we can see that squishy baby and add it to our pile of things that make us smile on the hard days.

SHOULD I RUSH TO THE HOSPITAL IF MY BAG OF WATER BROKE BUT I'M NOT HAVING CONTRACTIONS?

I do want to clarify that what I am about to say here is for term pregnancies only. If you are preterm, it's definitely important to get in touch with your obstetric provider, who will likely have you come in immediately for evaluation. How this is managed—potentially trying to stop labor, preventing infection, and figuring out why your bag of water broke so early—is very different from when your bag of water breaks when it's supposed to!

The bag of water breaking as the first sign of labor happens in about 8 percent of term (37 weeks or more) pregnancies. This is called prelabor rupture of membranes (PROM). With no contractions in sight, you might wonder if you need to immediately call your doctor or midwife and head into Labor and Delivery, or if you should hang out at home until you start to have contractions.

In general, OB-GYNs recommend that once your bag of water is broken, you make your way in to see us. We say this because it means that your baby is on the way (even if it doesn't feel like it yet) and the protective barrier that was once there to decrease infection risk is gone, so we'd like to get you and your baby checked out. It's not a run-the-red-lights situation by any means, though, so you shouldn't feel like you need to drop everything and run.

It's also perfectly OK to call your doctor or midwife if you'd like to be at home for a bit or you're not sure. They can talk through their thoughts about your particular history, rule out if there are concerns like meconium (more on page 123, "Should I be worried about meconium in my amniotic fluid?") or bleeding, and review the risks and benefits of waiting (more on that in the table below).

Once you do arrive and it is confirmed that your bag of water has broken, your team will check your baby's heart rate, assess for any signs of infection, put you on a monitor to see if you're having any contractions that you may not be feeling yet, and do the usual admission steps (see page 86, "What happens when I get admitted?").

Your doctor or midwife will then discuss the options for what to do next in terms of your labor management if you're still not feeling any contractions—that is, should they help labor along or let nature take its course? I review those choices below, with the caveat that the quality of studies that found many of the outcomes mentioned here wasn't great:

	Potential benefits	**Potential risks**	**Dr. Jen's thoughts**
Do nothing and wait for contractions to start on their own (also called **expectant management**)	Can feel more natural.	Increased risk of infection in the uterus and your baby. These risks increase the longer your bag of water has been broken and the more cervical exams you have.	• Labor usually starts on its own within twelve to twenty-four hours in almost everyone, so if you want to wait (as long as everything appears reassuring) after you've been counseled, it's definitely a choice. • It's also OK to choose a timeline that feels good for you—for example, seeing if anything happens in six or eight hours. • If you are GBS positive, however, waiting is *not* usually recommended.

	Potential benefits	Potential risks	Dr. Jen's thoughts
Give medicine to start contractions (also called **active management** or **inducing labor**)	· Shorter time in labor and in the hospital · Lower rates of uterine infection · Lower rates of infection and need for antibiotics to be given to your baby · Does *not* change your chances of needing a C-section	May feel more medicalized	In studies, those who chose induction for PROM viewed their experiences more positively than those who waited. (I found that tidbit interesting!)

The choice is always yours (as you'll hear me say many times in this book!), but in general the people who are truly best suited to going the expectant route are those who:

- Have a low-risk pregnancy
- Are GBS negative
- Have clear amniotic fluid
- Show no signs of infection
- Do not have vaginal bleeding
- Have no concerns about the baby's heart rate or growth
- Want to avoid cervical exams

I want you to remember **there is no clock that starts ticking once your bag of water breaks, where you must have your baby within twenty-four hours, or you have to have a C-section.** The latter is an outdated way of practicing, so if you're told that, feel free to speak up.

WHAT HAPPENS WHEN I GO TO TRIAGE TO GET CHECKED OUT?

The unknown can be scary, so I want to break down what a visit to labor and delivery triage looks like. Every unit may flow a bit differently, but this should work as a general idea.

1. You'll go directly to Labor and Delivery (L&D) or be told to check into the Emergency Department (ED); sometimes it depends on the time of day. Most EDs have a cutoff around 18 to 20 weeks of pregnancy, and once you're past that, you automatically get taken to L&D to be evaluated. They'll help get you up there (and quickly, because in general they are deathly afraid of pregnant people).
2. You'll let the front desk secretary know the reason for your visit, and you'll be shown to a room. In general, triage rooms are smaller than the room you'll be in once you're admitted for labor, so don't worry if it seems woefully tiny.
3. Your triage nurse will ask why you've come in and will get some more details so that they can relay this to the obstetric provider. They'll often have you change into a hospital gown and provide a urine sample before getting your vital signs and hooking you up to the monitors that check your baby's heart rate and your uterine activity.
4. If you come in because you think you're in labor, the nurse will check your cervix (though at some hospitals, such as those with residents, they may hold off on doing this and have the provider do it). If you think your water broke, they will do a speculum exam and perform a few tests to see if it has (with the same caveat as above).

Curious about how many cervical exams you can expect? Head to page 117, "How often will they check my cervix?"

5. After this, they will leave the room to call the obstetric provider who will be seeing you. It may be a resident, midwife, OB hospitalist, or your doctor, who may be at home or in the hospital (more on page 4, which describes different models of care).

6. A provider may come and chat with you right away and/or examine you. Or if it's clear you're in labor or your water broke, they will admit you to Labor and Delivery. If your doctor or midwife is at home, they may order some tests or monitoring over the phone and only come in when those results are back, or it may just be the nurse who physically sees you the entire time.

7. If you came in for a labor check and it's not clear if it's time, you may have a repeat cervical exam in a few hours to help determine if you're in labor. During this time, you may be monitored continuously, or you may be taken off the monitors—it depends on your pregnancy and how your baby has looked while on the monitor so far.

8. If it's determined you're not yet in active labor or your water hasn't broken, your team will likely recommend that you be discharged and go back home. If your contractions are painful, though, they may recommend some medicine to help you get some rest.

9. Prior to you going home, they'll give instructions for warning signs and reasons to return. You can ask as many questions as you like to make sure you feel informed and comfortable with the plan.

If you are worried that you're being sent home too soon or you're not being heard, you can and should voice your concerns. I've got you covered in the next section on how to navigate this.

WHAT IF I GET SENT HOME FROM TRIAGE BUT SOMETHING DOESN'T FEEL RIGHT?

You shouldn't leave the hospital feeling less certain than when you came in, because the point is to get answers and have a plan you feel confident in. I know that's unfortunately not always the case, though.

Here are some suggestions if you feel like you're not being heard, or you think you're being sent home too early:

1. **Ask to get another opinion.** Maybe you think the person who checked your cervix wasn't sure of themselves, or you just feel like another set of eyes on your case would help. You can do this by saying something like, "Is there any way you can run this by another provider here? I'm feeling like another person's input on this would help me feel confident in this plan, or have other ideas that I might feel better about."

2. **Ask to be given a few more hours.** Your cervix may not have dilated more over two hours, but it doesn't mean we're 100 percent sure you're not in active labor. If you're still super uncomfortable or worried because you live far from the hospital and a repeat trip back will be difficult, you can certainly ask for a little more time before being sent home. Or maybe you've been told your bag of water hasn't broken but you really think it has; you can always ask for another evaluation in an hour to see if the results are different.

3. **Go up the chain.** If you've voiced your concerns and you're brushed off, you can ask to speak to the charge nurse, nurse manager, and/or patient advocate. I know you might be worried about being labeled difficult, but you deserve to be heard. Ways to phrase this could be:

    - I am concerned I am not being heard. Can I please speak to someone else?
    - I am uncomfortable with this plan. Who can I talk to about this?

- I am worried me going home now is a safety issue for me and my baby. Who is the right person to address this?

4. **Get evaluated somewhere else.** The good news is that this isn't often needed, but if you are sent home from triage and something doesn't feel right, as a last resort you can always be seen at another hospital. This isn't convenient, and in some places where other hospitals aren't within driving distance this might not be an option—but if it is for you, you can do this. Be honest about why you've come to this second hospital, as this helps inform them as to where you're coming from (and, truthfully, most electronic records are accessible everywhere, so they'd likely see notes from your prior visit to the other hospital).
5. **Go home, but return if things don't get better or they worsen.** Sometimes we really think baby isn't coming, so we send you home, only to have you return four hours later in full-blown active labor. I always tell my patients that our tests and our protocols are good but not perfect, so returning if your gut tells you something is wrong is more than OK.

WHAT IF I WANT TO GO HOME TO LABOR FOR A WHILE AND THEN COME BACK? CAN I DO THAT?

You're always the one in charge of your body, so I'd say yes—but also please consider the recommendations of your healthcare team.

For someone with a low-risk pregnancy who is seen in triage and is clearly in the earlier stage of labor, wanting to go home and come back in when things level up is not a bad idea at all. This allows you to be in your own environment with the option to come in when you feel ready. The downside of this is that if you can't make it back in time, you might birth at home (less common if it's your first) or by the time you arrive you might miss the chance for an epidural if that's what you're wanting.

If you've got any high-risk issues, like high blood pressure, or if your baby's heart rate tracing has us concerned, going home might not be something we recommend. If this is the case for you, ask us why we want you to stay so that you can be fully informed. A good compromise might be that you stay on Labor and Delivery but we minimize disturbing you in your room, dim the lights, and do whatever we can to give you a homelike environment with the privacy you desire.

At the end of the day, we can never force you to stay, but if we see something concerning and it would be against our medical advice for you to leave, we may have you sign a form that states you acknowledge these risks. Yes, it's mostly to cover us legally, but also to document that we really did have a thorough discussion. If this is your situation, know that you can (and we want you to!) come back at any time.

WHAT DO I DO IF I GO PAST MY DUE DATE?

I went two days past my due date with my second and I thought he'd never come out (he did, and yes, I realize I was being rather dramatic).

The bad news: Only 5 percent of babies are born on their due date.

The good news: I promise you won't be pregnant forever.

Therefore, I want to remind you that a due date is an estimate. In medical terms we call it your EDD, or *estimated* delivery date. It's right there in the name, but I know from personal experience that it's hard not to see it as a guarantee.

With that in mind, knowing the terms below is important, because it helps understand why we might recommend inducing your labor versus waiting for nature to take its course:

- **Early-term pregnancy:** 37 weeks 0 days to 38 weeks 6 days
- **Full-term pregnancy:** 39 weeks 0 days through 40 weeks 6 days

- **Late-term pregnancy:** 41 weeks 0 days to 41 weeks 6 days
- **Post-term pregnancy:** 42 weeks 0 days and beyond (thankfully, only about 5 percent of babies wait it out this long)

So here's what is generally recommended if that due date sails on by:

	Additional monitoring (fetal heart rate and ultrasound monitoring)	Induction of labor
40 weeks 0 days–40 weeks 6 days	Not recommended	Optional
41 weeks 0 days–41 weeks 6 days	Recommended	Optional
42 weeks 0 days and after	If not induced, recommended	Recommended

In general, we don't recommend pregnancy going past 42 weeks. This is because data shows us that this increases your risk of a large baby, of your baby having their first poop in the uterus and breathing it in (meconium aspiration), of low amniotic fluid (oligohydramnios, which can lead to heart rate issues in labor, as the umbilical cord can get squished), having a C-section, and stillbirth.

I want to dive into **stillbirth** more. This is a tragic outcome and something that is usually the main reason your provider may discuss an induction labor once you hit 41 weeks of pregnancy. This is because the risk increases after 37 weeks, but most notably after 41 weeks. Thankfully, the overall risk is still rather small, but given how terrible it is, we do pay attention to it.

Gestational age	Stillbirth risk (per 1,000 pregnancies)	Stillbirth risk as a percentage
37 weeks	0.21	0.02%
42 weeks	1.08	0.11%

Put another way, based on a study out of the United Kingdom:

For pregnancies that continue . . .	This number of extra stillbirths and newborn deaths	Stillbirth risk as a percentage
From 40 to 41 weeks	1.66 more per 1,000 pregnancies	0.17%
From 41 to 42 weeks	3.18 more per 1,000 pregnancies	0.32%

It's ultimately your decision if these numbers feel unacceptably high to risk continuing your pregnancy or not. They also need to be taken in the context of other issues that may be at play in your pregnancy, such as whether you have diabetes, whether ultrasound indicates your baby has stopped growing, or whether the placenta looks calcified (an indicator it's not functioning that well anymore). Whether or not to induce your labor based on your due date should take into account any other pregnancy risk factors, your baby's monitoring and amniotic fluid levels, and shared decision-making between you and your provider (not the TikTok "For You" page).

OK, BUT HOW CAN I MAKE MY BABY COME OUT?

The good news is that you don't have to feel helpless if your due date comes and goes. Good data shows that **membrane sweeping,** which is where during a cervical exam we use a finger to gently separate the bag of water from the lower part of the uterus, can make it less likely you'll still be pregnant by 41 weeks. While it doesn't always work, it can be repeated (though the optimal frequency still remains to be determined), and we estimate that **one induction of labor is avoided for every eight pregnant people who have this done.** Side effects can include pain during the sweep, cramping or contractions (which is actually the point), your bag of water breaking, and vaginal bleeding.

I always get asked about the other ways to help bring on labor, such as having sex and all the other unsolicited things your family and friends are "helpfully" suggesting. Here is the evidence:

Method	Data
Nipple stimulation	Has been shown to work if your cervix is already dilated, but ask your provider first if this is safe for you to try.
Eating dates	Studies show eating dates in the third trimester may shorten pregnancy length and decrease the need for an induction. Optimal quantities are not known, and the data is not of the highest quality, but the chance of harm is very low. Do be sure to check in with your provider if you have diabetes, however, as the sugar content may not make this intervention a good option for you.
Having sex	No data to support, or data shows it doesn't help.
Walking	No data to support, or data shows it doesn't help.
Castor oil	No data to support, or data shows it doesn't help. Castor oil may make you vomit.
Teas and tinctures	No data to support, or data shows it doesn't help.
Acupressure	No data to support, or data shows it doesn't help.
Acupuncture	*May* help with cervical ripening (i.e., softening and preparation for labor), but the data is limited.

My take? Feel free to try these things (except the castor oil, because you'll just puke) if they feel right for you, but it's perfectly fine to skip them, too.

WELCOME TO THE (BIRTHDAY) PARTY

DOCTOR DOULA

I was caring for a patient once who was all by herself while in labor with her second baby. She unfortunately had no support people present, so we all jumped in and rallied around her as best we could. This was an all-hands-on-deck situation—she was in active labor and was opting for an unmedicated birth.

There was a good amount of screaming. We heard lots of unsavory words. As she grabbed and squeezed my hands during her contractions, I remember worrying whether I'd be able to use them to operate later. For the most part, a pretty typical day on Labor and Delivery, but still—it kept us on our toes!

After about an hour she requested (emphatically) an epidural. I asked if I could check her cervix, as I thought she might be close to delivering, and she said yes. When I let her know that she was 8 centimeters dilated, I told her the rest of the dilation might occur too quickly for an epidural, or if she did get it, it might not kick in quickly enough—but we could definitely try if she wanted it. She let us know she wanted it no matter what, so we called the anesthesia resident who was on call to come to the room now.

Minutes later he was there and was all in for trying to get this mom the break she so desperately wanted. It took a few moments to place the epidural, as it was hard for her to sit still enough, but finally it was in.

Then she lay down to try to help the medicine distribute evenly in her body . . . and that's when I saw that this epidural wasn't going to have the chance to work.

"*The baby is coming now!*" she cried.

The anesthesia resident was trapped up at the head of her bed, as his equipment and my delivery cart were blocking his escape.

What he did next, I will never forget: Rather than trying to run out of there at all costs (like many a non-obstetric doctor would do, and

I wouldn't blame them), he grabbed her hand when she reached for him. He told her to breathe and that it was going to be OK. Moments later, when she delivered her baby, he lit up with excitement as he said, "You did it! You were so amazing!" He was the one who took their first family photos, making sure to get every angle.

When we were all finished and left the room, he had a huge smile on his face. "I never really get to be in the room when it's like that! It was crazy! And so cool!" Everyone at the nurses' station laughed. After that, we gave him the nickname of Dr. Doula—which, to our delight, he proudly embraced.

I love this story because it was such a stark reminder that what I get to do every day (and night) really is the coolest job in the world. And that support can come from so many beautiful, unexpected places.

WHAT ARE THE REASONS I CAN GET ADMITTED TO LABOR AND DELIVERY?

I already covered some of this on page 50, "How do I know when to go to the hospital?" Of course, "When you're in labor!" is one answer. But that's not the only reason your doctor or midwife might say it's time to stay.

Keep in mind that you might be admitted to the hospital, but it doesn't mean you're having your baby. Your team may want to watch you to get more information before making any decisions. This means you might get sent home with a baby still in your uterus as opposed to in your arms. Your team will take into consideration why they are keeping you, how you and your baby are doing, and how far along you are. Not sure what the plan is or it's not making sense? Don't be afraid to speak up and ask!

This isn't a full list, but the most common reasons to be admitted are:

1. When you are in active labor. Active labor is defined as being 6 centimeters dilated, but you can absolutely be on the active labor train if you're less than 6 centimeters and are also having regular, painful contractions with a cervix that's thinning out. So don't take this to mean that 6 centimeters is the magic number—it's but one part of a larger picture.
2. Your bag of water has broken.
3. You're having bleeding that is more than we can write off to your cervix dilating or bloody show (the bloody, mucusy, snot-like discharge that can be seen when your cervix is preparing for labor).
4. Your baby is showing signs that he or she isn't loving being in the uterus anymore, as seen in certain kinds of heart rate tracing patterns (I go into this more on page 95, "Talk to me about fetal monitoring").
5. You've had an ultrasound that has diagnosed concerns regarding your baby's growth, low amniotic fluid, or poor placental blood flow.
6. You've been diagnosed with something that makes staying pregnant too risky for you or your baby, such as preeclampsia or an infection in the uterus.

7. You've gone well past your due date (for more on this, see page 63, "What do I do if I go past my due date?").

8. You're admitted to get medication to help you rest and deal with painful contractions while seeing if you really are in active labor. This is often called therapeutic rest, and the goal is to help you get some relief while we see if your contractions will stall out or not. Sometimes this looks like an overnight admission, with the possibility of going home in the morning if contractions settle down and your cervix doesn't change.

MY DOCTOR WANTS TO INDUCE MY LABOR. SHOULD I?

Let me be clear that inductions are neither all good nor all bad: They are a tool that has a time and a place. Used correctly, they can be lifesaving. Carried out improperly or when not needed, they can lead to an increase in C-sections, other interventions, and babies born too soon who may need to go to the NICU. And with almost one in three births in 2020 involving an induction of labor, it's worth going into this conversation with all the info you need to make an informed choice.

Here are some scenarios when staying pregnant may be riskier to you or your baby than undergoing an induction. (Big caveat: There are lots of gray areas here and individual circumstances that need to be considered, but I hope this is a helpful starting point for understanding why your doc or midwife may be having the induction conversation.)

Pregnancy complication	Why induction might be recommended
Severe preeclampsia	This kind of preeclampsia can be deadly. Once you reach a certain point in your pregnancy, your team may recommend induction to avoid risks of stroke, heart attacks, and other complications. More about this complication on page 155, "I was told I have high blood pressure and I'm scared."
Your bag of water has broken early	If you're preterm and your bag of water broke, there is a risk of infection and placental abruption. Your team will likely recommend an induction once you are around 34 to 35 weeks of pregnancy (though potentially earlier if they are worried, or later if all is stable), once the risk of an ongoing pregnancy outweighs the benefit of allowing your baby to continue to grow and develop.
Your baby isn't growing normally, or has abnormally low amniotic fluid	It might sound weird that your doctor recommends an induction if your baby is very small (you may hear the term **IUGR,** or intrauterine growth restriction) or there isn't enough amniotic fluid—shouldn't the baby stay in and grow? The opposite is true, however: When we see signs that the placenta is not working well, it means your baby is at risk of not growing at all, which could lead to fetal distress and stillbirth.
You have diabetes in pregnancy or high blood pressure	Depending on how well controlled these are and whether you are on medicines for them, your providers may recommend an induction before your due date.
Your medical conditions	If you've got worsening lung or heart issues or need to undergo a treatment that might not be safe in pregnancy, your team may recommend you deliver early.
Issues in the uterus such as an infection (chorioamnionitis) or bleeding (such as from placental abruption)	Both issues can become serious rather quickly, and an induction may be recommended. However, if they are truly life-threatening, your team may suggest a C-section instead.

Pregnancy complication	Why induction might be recommended
You're pregnant with more than one baby	Depending on how many babies there are and the type of multiples (more on page 173, "What happens differently for twins? Triplets?"), delivery will be recommended earlier than your due date.
You go past your due date	Head to page 63, "What do I do if I go past my due date?," for info on what to do if your due date passes you by. Your provider may recommend induction to decrease the risk of stillbirth and other complications.

I want to reiterate once more that a recommendation for induction should be a conversation and shared decision between you and your doctor or midwife. It's rarely one-size-fits-all, so if you aren't clear on why it's being offered, feel free to ask the following:

1. Why are you recommending an induction? Why at this time in my pregnancy, and not a different date?
2. What are the alternatives? Is choosing to do more frequent monitoring a safe option?
3. What are the risks to me and my baby with an induction? Or with staying pregnant longer?
4. If I am induced now, what are the chances my baby will need to go to the NICU? Would they need to be transferred to a different hospital?
5. Am I able to get another opinion?

To clarify that last point especially: You can always ask for another opinion if you are concerned, but know that another opinion may not always be available depending on where you live, your access to care, and the acuity of the situation.

On the flip side, these are some red flags if your doctor or midwife recommends an induction:

The reason given	Dr. Jen's thoughts
Your doctor is going out of town.	If this is the only person in town who can deliver your baby, that's one thing—but quite another if one of their partners could be there for your birth!
To get your baby delivered before a holiday.	Need I say more?
"I induce all my patients."	No.

And lastly, the gray areas:

The reason given	Dr. Jen's thoughts
You live far from the hospital.	If you live two hours or more from the closest hospital and have a history of rapid labors, this could be a reasonable option.
Your baby is measuring big, so this is to prevent them from getting bigger.	I know this sounds like it makes sense, but studies disagree on whether inducing you prevents complications from having a bigger baby, like a shoulder dystocia (see page 168, "What is a shoulder dystocia?") or needing a C-section. Currently, there is no evidence this should be done before 38 completed weeks of pregnancy, and after that it's *definitely* an individualized decision.
"Haven't you heard of the ARRIVE trial? Because of it, I offer inductions to all my patients at 39 weeks."	More than I can fit in this box—see the next section!

This was *a lot* about inductions of labor. Part of me wants to apologize, but the other part of me wants you to have all the information at your fingertips so you and your provider can make the best plan for you and your baby.

Take-home message: Most inductions without a medical reason should not happen until you hit 39 weeks, so that your baby has enough time to grow and develop.

MY DOCTOR SAYS A TRIAL SHOWED IT'S SAFEST TO GIVE BIRTH AT 39 WEEKS, SO SHOULD I BE INDUCED THEN?

This is your doctor referencing the ARRIVE trial. "ARRIVE" stands for "A Randomized Trial of Induction Versus Expectant Management," and this was a trial that was done in the United States in 2018 that included about 6,000 participants and was designed to answer a question about inducing labor. It looked at electively inducing healthy first-time pregnant people once they were 39 weeks.

There's a lot of misunderstanding about what the trial was and how we should use it to impact pregnancy care, so here are the talking points you need:

- **What they compared:** One group that had an elective induction at 39 weeks versus one group that waited for labor to start on its own.
- **What they found in the induced group:**

Benefits for mom	Benefits for baby
Decreased C-section rate (from 22.2% to 18.6%)	Decreased need for help breathing (from 4% to 3%)
Decreased rate of high blood pressure/ preeclampsia (from 14% to 9%)	

- **What they *didn't* find:**
  - Being induced did *not* decrease the risk of stillbirth.
  - It did not increase the risk of bad outcomes in the people being induced, but follow-up studies have shown mixed results (with some showing a small *increased* risk of blood transfusions, infections, and ICU admission in the induced group).
- **Key point of the study:** They used *very* specific induction protocols. This means they didn't give up on an induction too quickly (it can take a while; see page 78, "I've been told I need an induction of labor—how long does this take?"). If they hadn't done this, there likely would have been *more* C-sections in the group that was induced.

So, my thoughts on the ARRIVE trial and being told an induction at 39 weeks is your safest bet:

1. It can certainly be an option.
2. Some benefits are there, but they aren't so dramatic that this trial made us doctors say, "This data is amazing! We *must* induce all our patients at 39 weeks or else!"
3. This study only included low-risk first-timers. You can't assume this data applies to you if you're not in that group.
4. If you choose induction, you need to know it means interventions—we can't do inductions without medications and procedures. If you want a hands-off approach, this is not for you.
5. If you go for it, you need to clarify with your team that they are all in and aren't going to throw in the towel too quickly and thus commit you to a C-section.
6. Your hospital's labor and delivery unit may not be staffed to handle elective inductions, so they may not even be allowed to schedule them.

7. Even if you do schedule an elective induction, you may get "bumped" by people with medical issues.

8. **As with all things, this is ultimately up to you and should be a decision you make with your doctor or midwife and your individual situation and goals.**

I'VE BEEN TOLD I NEED AN INDUCTION OF LABOR—HOW LONG DOES THIS TAKE?

I won't lie: It really can feel like years.

An induction of labor—where we try to get your body to go into labor before it does on its own—can take days for some people. This might seem excessive, but as long as you and your baby are doing OK, then it's perfectly safe. In fact, us throwing in the towel too early before trying all our methods could mean an unnecessary C-section for you, which makes your next pregnancy a bit riskier. We really do need to focus on patience and giving things time to work.

The hardest scenario I often see with inductions is a feeling that nothing is working or happening. This often comes from friends or family members who keep texting and asking some version of "Is he here yet?" or "Is this healthy for the baby?" or "Wow! My induction only took eight hours!" So fun.

If your cervix isn't "ripe"—meaning it's not yet dilated or shortened that much—then methods to ripen it are the first part of an induction. It's normal for this to take hours to even a day or so (more on this in the next section). If it's your first baby, or if you're very preterm and we really have to convince your uterus that it truly is time to get active, the induction process can be sloooow. And that's normal and expected.

BUT WHAT IF IT SEEMS TO BE TAKING TOO LONG—LIKE, *WAY* TOO LONG?

Head to page 127, "They say my labor is going too slowly—what does that mean?," for information on when we start to get concerned about a lengthy labor. It's important to remember, however, that inductions are on a totally different timeline than spontaneous labor.

Let me introduce you to a term I despise: "failed induction of labor." I dislike any terminology that links failure to pregnancy or birth, but I'm telling you about it in case you hear it. Maybe knowing this is considered a medical term (and not a personal one) can take some of the sting out of it if you see it on your chart.

Current recommendations say that a C-section for a failed induction shouldn't be done until it's been twelve to eighteen hours after your bag of water is broken *and* you've been on Pitocin to bring on active labor—and potentially longer in certain scenarios. This means inductions can take time, and sometimes patience is our best tool here. The opposite can also be true, though, as when your medical stability or that of your baby doesn't allow your team to wait that long.

And once more on the term "failed": I hate it. I am only using it because that's what you might hear.

Here are some questions you can ask if your provider is suggesting your induction isn't working:

1. Am I in latent or active labor?
2. If I'm in latent labor, have I been given twelve to eighteen hours on Pitocin after my water broke? If not, why not? Do we have time to try that?
3. Is there something you are concerned about that makes a C-section our best course, or do we have time to wait a little longer?

One of the best ways to get through a longer induction is to rest when you can, even though I know you're excited. So often I see people who have lots of visitors from the very start and so they miss this chance to rest before things get intense. Then when the time to push comes along, they are truly exhausted. You can ask your team for updates, their input on the process, and when they think you should assemble the troops closer to your baby's arrival.

And maybe put your phone on Do Not Disturb.

HOW DOES AN INDUCTION WORK?

No two inductions are the same, but there are some general guidelines, and if you know those going into your induction, you will be super prepared. This section has lots of info—as I mentioned in the previous section, with one in three labors being induced, I want you to have *all* the info you might need.

First up: I can't stress enough that **it is normal for inductions of labor to sometimes take days.** I go into this in more detail in the next section, but know that if you are starting with an unfavorable cervix (more below), this can be *very* normal!

There are two basic pathways: (1) your cervix is checked → it gets a score → cervical ripening (if needed) is done, and (2) straight to induction.

Your cervix is checked

With two fingers we check your cervix not only to see how open or dilated it is, but also how much it has thinned out (reported as a percentage from zero to 100 percent), where it's positioned (front/middle/back), how low your baby is in the pelvis, and how it feels (soft, medium, or firm). We assign a score based on these findings to give you something called a **Bishop score:**

If your score is . . .	**Your cervix is considered . . .**	**Which means . . .**	**And your provider will . . .**
0 to 6	Unfavorable/unripe	Your cervix is not yet ready for contractions (because it would be like pushing against a closed door). Instead, it needs to be "ripened," which means providing help to soften and thin the cervix and slightly open the door.	Recommend cervical ripening either via medicine or mechanically (more below)
7 to 13	Favorable/ripe	It's ready for labor!	Start your induction with medicine to get your contractions going and/or break your bag of water

Let's get that cervix ripe

Yes, we really do talk about your cervix like a fruit, and no, I am not sure I love it either. But think of an unripe banana versus a ripe one—a softer, riper one peels (opens) easier, just like your cervix!

Here are the most common ways we ripen your cervix during an induction:

Method	How it's used	How it works	Pros	Cons	Dr. Jen's notes
Misoprostol (Cytotec)	Small pills that can be placed vaginally, taken by mouth, or placed under the tongue and dissolved, usually every four hours	Contains medicine similar to hormones in your body that soften and thin the cervix and cause it to open slightly. It can cause contractions, but often not as many as in active labor.	· Very inexpensive · Works the same as or better than Cervidil	· Can cause something called tachysystole (too many uterine contractions), which sometimes leads to concerning heart rate tracings · Can't be used if you're already contracting too much · Usually can't be fully removed once it is placed in the vagina · Can't be used if you've had a C-section (in most scenarios)	Misoprostol can work really well and can be given over multiple doses if needed. This is also the same medicine we use to treat bleeding after pregnancy as well as for spontaneous and induced abortions, so we are very comfortable using it.
Dinoprostone (Cervidil)	This is an insert (think of a small tampon) that is placed in the vagina until active labor begins, up to a maximum of twelve hours		Can be removed from the vagina if your baby isn't tolerating the medicine	· Expensive—not all hospitals carry it · Can't be used if you've had a C-section (in most scenarios)	I may be biased because it's expensive, but this is never my first go-to when it comes to cervical ripening.

Method	How it's used	How it works	Pros	Cons	Dr. Jen's notes
Cervical catheter (sometimes called cervical balloon/bulb or Foley balloon/bulb)	A catheter tube is placed through the cervix and filled with saline, then taped to tension on your leg. It usually falls out once your cervix is 3–4 centimeters dilated. It is usually removed after twelve hours if it hasn't fallen out on its own.	This mechanically dilates the cervix because of the pressure of the filled balloon against the cervix.	• Can be used if you've had a C-section • Can be placed even if you're having contractions • Can be used in combination with misoprostol or Pitocin • Some providers place this in clinic. You then go home and come back the next day or when it comes out, thus decreasing your time in the hospital.	• Placement can be painful for some people • Placement isn't always possible if your cervix is closed or hard to reach	While the insertion is usually very quick (just a few minutes), if it's painful don't hesitate to ask for pain medicine to make it more comfortable. This can be a great way to ripen a cervix, especially if you've had a C-section before.

Note: There are some other methods of cervical ripening, but these are the most common ones used today.

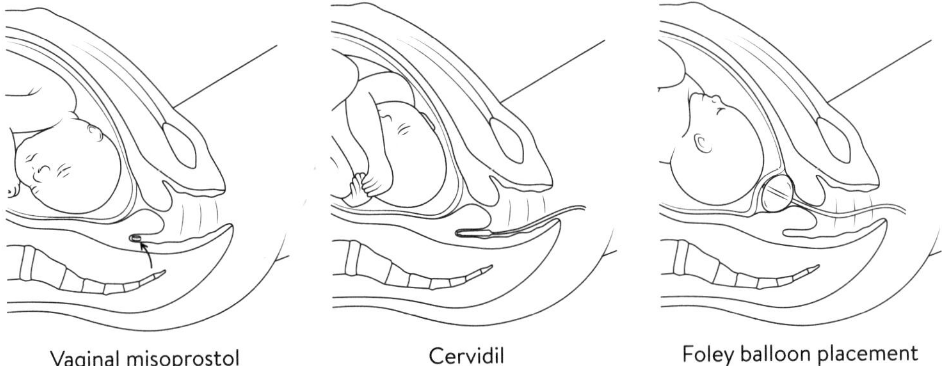

Vaginal misoprostol

Cervidil

Foley balloon placement

Ripe and ready to go

Once your cervix is ready for labor, we can help bring on contractions and get you into active labor using the following methods. Most inductions include a combination of a few techniques—there really is no one recipe for induction that works for everyone.

Method	How it's used	How it works	Pros	Cons	Dr. Jen's notes
Pitocin	A continuous drip via your IV. It can be dosed up or down with the goal of getting you to contract regularly every few minutes.	This is a synthetic form of the hormone oxytocin, which your body makes.	• Works very well in causing contractions • The dose can be adjusted to what your body needs—it's not one-size-fits-all • Can be stopped if needed	For risks, see page 124, "What is Pitocin and why might they suggest I need it?"	It's almost a guarantee if your labor is induced that this will be used at some point.
Breaking your bag of water	During a cervical exam, we use a small hook (either at the end of something that looks like a crochet needle or on our finger) to break the bag of water.	This causes the release of hormones that can lead to contractions. It also leads to more pressure of your baby's head on the cervix, which also helps the cervix to dilate.	• Often very easy to do • Can be an effective method combined with Pitocin to shorten labor • Allows for the placement of internal monitors if needed (see page 98, "And they want to put monitors . . . inside of me?")	If you're GBS positive, we usually want you to have antibiotics for this before we break your bag. See page 118, "I was told I'm GBS positive and I'm freaking out," and page 121, "My doctor wants to break my bag of water and I'm not sure if I should."	In case you're worried, the bag of water doesn't have nerve fibers, so this does not hurt! You will continue to leak fluid during your labor, and yes, it feels like you're peeing yourself.

Method	How it's used	How it works	Pros	Cons	Dr. Jen's notes
Membrane stripping or sweeping	During a cervical exam we run our fingers between the bag of water and the cervix to separate them.	This causes the release of hormones that can lead to contractions.	Can be done at your prenatal visits once you are at term to help bring on spontaneous labor	• Can be crampy and cause some bleeding • Not usually used as a stand-alone way to induce labor once you're in the hospital	I love a good membrane sweep once you're full term! This can also be repeated, with data to support that it can help you go into labor within forty-eight hours and decrease your need for a hospital induction.
Nipple stimulation	Your hands, a nursing baby, or a breast pump is used to stimulate one breast at a time.	Just like with breastfeeding, this causes the release of oxytocin, a hormone that causes milk letdown as well as uterine contractions.	• Pretty easy and cheap to do! • Hasn't been shown to cause issues in the low-risk pregnancies that were studied	• Some hospitals may be uncomfortable with you doing this because they may not have a protocol for how to do it. • One way to do it is to pump one breast for fifteen minutes, then switch to the other, for a total of an hour. Stop when you start to contract every few minutes or if nothing is happening after one hour.	If you're doing this at home, check with your provider to make sure they're aware and on board (it's only been studied in low-risk pregnancies). Tends to work best when your cervix is already ripe. Not recommended before you are full term (39 weeks pregnant or more).

Note: There are other ways to induce labor that tend to be used in homebirths/birth centers, such as herbs. These are not generally used in the hospital, so I will not be covering them here.

DR. JEN'S TOP TIPS FOR INDUCTIONS OF LABOR

1. **Bring all the things to keep you entertained.** Books, shows to stream, snacks, games—all of it. This can help make the time go by more quickly.
2. **Try to sleep when you can.** The worst thing is to be awake for forty-eight hours only to have to push for three hours on zero sleep. Bring an eye mask and a white-noise machine or phone app, and don't hesitate to ask for medicine to help you sleep if you need to.
3. **Tell friends and family *you'll* call *them*.** Nothing makes you feel more like a watched pot than everyone texting asking what's taking so long.
4. **Have fair expectations.** Know that it can take a while. That's OK! Your body spent months keeping that baby in, so it's normal for it to need some convincing to change course.
5. **Don't brag to your friends if it goes super fast.** Or they'll get really mad at us when the same isn't true for them!

WHAT HAPPENS WHEN I GET ADMITTED?

Here's a quick rundown of what it can look like to get admitted to Labor and Delivery when the plan is for you to have your baby. Of course, a given hospital might do things a bit differently, but in general you can expect the following:

1. After being seen by the nurse or obstetric provider and the decision has been made for you to be admitted, the team caring for you will

contact your doctor or midwife (if they weren't the ones to initially evaluate you). They'll place orders to get the process going.

2. You may be **moved to a different room.** This new room may be a bit bigger and better equipped for labor.

3. You may be **assigned to a new nurse,** who will be introduced to you by the nurse you had for your initial evaluation. They will often go over with each other what's been done so far, why you're staying, and any relevant history. This often happens in the room with you so that you can answer any questions and be part of the conversation.

4. Your nurse will **place an IV** (more on this on page 102, "Do I really need an IV in my arm?") and draw blood for standard admission lab work. This can usually be done with the same poke to minimize discomfort. Sometimes a person who specializes in IV placement will do this if your nurse is struggling or if you're known to be a hard stick—speak up if this is the case! The bloodwork we usually order includes checking your blood count and platelets as well as your blood type (so that we can have some blood on hand in case a situation arises where we may recommend a transfusion). Additional tests may be ordered for your specific situation.

5. **You'll probably be asked *a lot* of admission questions,** ranging from your medical history and medications you take to what pediatrician you've picked and who your emergency contact is. It may seem like a lot, but it's done so that all your important info is up to date and confirmed by the people who'll be caring for you and your baby.

6. You'll **sign consents** to allow your team to treat you. This is pretty standard, but definitely feel free to ask questions.

7. You may be **placed on fetal monitoring** continuously or intermittently depending on your situation (more on this on page 95, "Talk to me about fetal monitoring"). You may also have a quick ultrasound done to confirm the position of your baby.

8. Your nurse will ask you **what your birth preferences are** for your labor and birth (and if they don't, I recommend you bring it up ASAP, since it's important). See page 44, "Should I make a birth plan . . . or does every OB-GYN hate them?," for more on things to consider and how this discussion can go.
9. If you're **having a C-section,** some additional things will happen, which I cover on page 129, "Talk to me about C-sections."

After that, it's off to the races! If at any point you are feeling like something isn't feeling right or you're not being heard, please speak up. I cover more on how to do this on page 138, "I don't feel I'm being listened to. What are my options?"

WHO ARE THE PEOPLE WHO WILL BE CARING FOR ME ON LABOR AND DELIVERY?

Birth is a team effort, and so you may have some or all of these folks at your labor and birthday party!

Your nursing team

This can include a primary nurse who is caring for you, but you will likely see more than one during a shift, as your primary nurse will need breaks to eat or pee (important things!). They often do twelve-hour shifts, so depending on how long your labor is you may have more than one main nurse. You may also be visited by the charge nurse, who is the nurse in charge of the unit.

Your obstetric team

OB-GYN, midwifery, and family medicine practices can be set up differently, so who is going to be caring for you on Labor and Delivery can vary—and why you should ask at your very first prenatal visit to make sure you're familiar with and OK with how your provider's team works.

Here are some potential models:

1. Your obstetric provider is not physically present. They are in clinic, the operating room, or at home and are a phone call away. Your nurse will call them with any updates and when it's time to have a baby. Often in these scenarios, your nurse will do most of the cervical exams and you'll see your provider when they come in to check on you (such as in between OR cases or when it's time to birth).
2. Your obstetric provider's group always has someone physically present on Labor and Delivery via shift work. This means you could see your doctor or midwife, or someone covering for their group. In these practice models, you'll often be visited by the OB-GYN and midwife more frequently since they are there on the unit. Some practices using this model have whoever is on Labor and Delivery that day deliver your baby; other practices will use the hospital provider to manage your labor but will call in your OB-GYN or midwife to be at your birth. You should clarify this so that you know what to expect!
3. You may be cared for by an OB hospitalist. This is an OB-GYN who works only in the hospital caring for patients who are pregnant or postpartum. This is what I do, and I love it! OB hospitalists are experts in managing emergency situations and are often the go-to doctors when another OB-GYN or midwife needs help, or if they are not present when one of their patients needs to be seen. **Data continues to show that having an OB hospitalist present on Labor and Delivery makes birth safer by decreasing the number of poor outcomes for birthing people and their babies.** If given the choice, I would always pick a hospital where I knew an OB hospitalist was going to be present 24/7.

Your pediatric team

In some hospitals, pediatricians employed by the hospital see and care for all babies born there. Others have an open policy, meaning community pediatricians can come in and see babies that they'll eventually be caring for in their practice. It's worth knowing which model your hospital has so you know who to expect (head to page 40 for more on what to ask your baby's prospective pediatrician, in "When should I pick a pediatrician?").

Some hospitals are also equipped with neonatal intensive care units that are staffed by doctors and nurses who can care for babies born early or who have complex medical needs. NICUs vary based on the level of care they provide, with some taking all babies and others that have limits based on a baby's gestational age and the severity of a baby's issues.

This means if your hospital doesn't have a NICU or one at a high enough level and your baby needs extra help, they may have to be transferred to a different hospital and thus be separated from you. Being in this field and seeing what I have—and being married to a pediatrician—has definitely biased me to only give birth in a place where the highest level of NICU care is available. However, this may not be an option if you live in a rural area.

Your anesthesia team

We love an anesthesiologist who can take the labor pain away if that's what you're asking for! Some hospitals have anesthesiologists (who are doctors) and nurse anesthetists (nurses with specialty training in anesthesia, who are always supervised by the anesthesiologist) physically present in the hospital. And for hospitals whose labor units are big enough, they may have a dedicated obstetric anesthesia team. Other hospitals may need to call in their anesthesiologist from home—this is often the case in smaller or rural hospitals. In this situation they are usually required to be available within thirty minutes, which might not be ideal if you need an emergency C-section, where minutes make a difference. It may also mean having to wait a short time if you want an epidural in labor.

You should definitely ask what the anesthesia situation is at the hospital you plan to deliver at. I'll share that I never would have birthed in a place that didn't always have a dedicated OB anesthesiologist physically present, but that's the OB hospitalist in me.

Those who are learning

OK, hear me out: **I think giving birth in a place where learners like residents, medical students, and nursing students are present is a fantastic idea**—because it means you're in a hospital that prioritizes education and evidence-based care. It also means more *really* smart people who are keeping an eye on you and your baby, and often these are the people who have the most time to spend with you and may even be the most empathetic. I know not everyone thinks that way and would prefer that fewer people be involved in their birth, but I do want to encourage you to mull it over.

You can always decline having a student present in your care, but I would call out that at academic centers, residents (doctors who've graduated from medical school and are now doing their specialty training in their chosen field, like OB-GYN) are crucial to the care you receive, and not having them involved may not be an option. If this concerns you, giving birth at an academic hospital may not be the right place for you.

All the helpers!

You may come across other people during your labor and birth who are there to help and make your birth experience safe and smooth. This can include nursing assistants, who often will check your vital signs and help the nursing team; surgical techs, who help the doctors during C-sections and other surgeries and procedures; lab folks, who may be the ones to draw your blood; food services people, who always love getting to see a new baby; social workers, who can offer resources; other medical specialists, who may be asked to consult if needed; housekeeping staff (always be nice to them—they are often the least-paid, but the work they do is among the most crucial to keeping the hospital running). And we can't forget about the lactation consultants! I'll cover that more on page 244, "Who can help me with breastfeeding?"

WILL MY DOCTOR OR MIDWIFE BE THE ONE TO SEE ME AND BE WITH ME THE ENTIRE LABOR?

Probably not—but don't freak out!

As I mentioned in the question above, a lot of this depends on how your doctor or midwife's practice is set up. But even if they are physically present on Labor and Delivery, it's important to remember they may have multiple patients they are caring for at the same time. They're also responsible for seeing and caring for the postpartum patients who've already birthed. And if they are an OB-GYN, it's possible they may also be getting called to the emergency department or elsewhere in the hospital to see patients.

That said, this means you'll probably be seeing a lot more of your nurse while in labor, and this is normal! Nurses are an integral part of the team and experts in the labor process. When it comes time to push, your provider may or may not be in the room with you the entire time; they may only come periodically and then stay when it's obvious you're about to birth.

In general, it can be said that if you're cared for by a midwife, then you're more likely to have them there for the entire time you are pushing (which can be minutes to hours). This might be because they have fewer high-risk patients that they also need to keep an eye on, but also because this tends to be part of midwifery philosophy overall. Don't count us OB-GYNs out, though—when time allows, I've loved getting to spend the entire pushing stage with my patients!

I do want to address longer labors and let you know that if you're in labor for a long time, your provider and nurse will likely change as their shift ends. Some of us do twelve-hour shifts, while others stay for a full twenty-four hours. And while it might be tempting to wish that we stayed just *a bit longer* to be there for your birth, keep in mind that sleep deprivation can make us unsafe to be at work. You definitely want someone who is awake and alert to be caring for you, even if they might be a new face to you!

WHAT IS NORMAL LABOR, ANYWAY?

Such a good question! I am including this so that you can be informed if your nurse or provider brings up that your labor *isn't* progressing normally and recommends an intervention to help it along, or if you just want to get an idea of the average length of things. Why? Because this helps you ask the right questions and be aware whether an intervention is being recommended a bit too soon or is truly justified.

First, let's review the stages of labor:

Stage 1. In this stage, the cervix starts opening to complete dilation, which is 10 centimeters. This stage is divided into two parts:

- **Latent labor.** The slow, early phase of cervical change (opening and thinning).
- **Active labor.** More active cervical change. In general, this starts at about 6 centimeters.

Stage 2. This is the pushing phase. It lasts from when your cervix is completely dilated to the birth of your baby.

Stage 3. The time from your baby's birth to the delivery of the placenta.

So how do we define what "normal" labor is? This is based on studies looking at how thousands of people in labor progressed. We used to use older guidelines from the 1950s, called the Friedman labor curve, but now have more updated data that (thankfully) more accurately reflects labor. When used, this updated curve can lead to a lower C-section rate because it has broadened the definition of what "normal" labor progression is.

	Normal length	Notes
Stage 1 **Latent labor (up to 6 cm)**	• How long this phase lasts depends on how dilated your cervix was to start with • Can last up to sixteen hours!	If your labor is being induced, this can be *much* longer and still be considered normal—more on induced labor on page 80, "How does an induction work?"
Stage 1 **Active labor (6 cm or more)**	• 0.5 to about 1 cm dilation per hour is considered normal OR • Slow but continued cervical dilation every four hours	What number baby and whether or not you have an epidural can affect this speed—more on page 127, "They say my labor is going too slowly—what does that mean?"
Stage 2 **Pushing**	• Less than three hours in someone who's having their first baby • Less than two hours in someone who has had a baby vaginally before • If you have an epidural, an extra hour of pushing in both groups can be normal	• While these durations are considered "normal," they are *not* hard-and-fast limits if progress is being made while pushing but it's taking longer. • On the flip side, if *no* progress is being made at all in shorter time periods, it is not needed to wait the full two to three hours to proceed with a C-section (more on page 127, "They say my labor is going too slowly—what does that mean?").

	Normal length	Notes
Stage 3 **Placental delivery**	Less than thirty minutes	This usually takes only a couple of minutes. More on this on page 213, "When (and how) does the placenta come out?"

TALK TO ME ABOUT FETAL MONITORING.

I have a lot to say, but I can sum it up by saying that electronic fetal monitoring (EFM) is the technology many obstetric providers love to hate but that we're stuck with, even though it doesn't always help us. This technology was developed in the 1960s with the goal of decreasing the rates of stillbirth, cerebral palsy, and brain injury in labor related to a baby getting too little oxygen during the labor process.

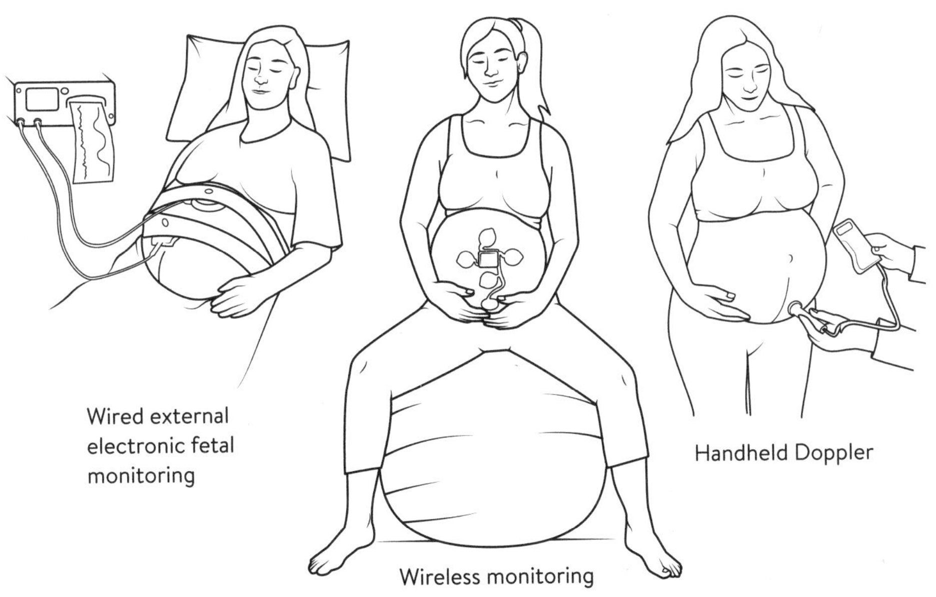

Wired external electronic fetal monitoring

Wireless monitoring

Handheld Doppler

While it *has* led to a small decrease in neonatal seizures after birth, it hasn't helped with the other poor outcomes it was meant to prevent. It has also led to an increase in C-section rates and the use of vacuum and forceps (more on these kinds of deliveries on page 193, "What is a vacuum or forceps, and why might I need it?").

Despite that, EFM is a technology that we use for basically all hospital births, my own birth included. We've got the medico-legal system and malpractice lawsuits to thank for that (as well as our own personal stories where we saw a terrible tracing, did an emergency C-section, and truly saved a baby's life—but I'd be lying if I didn't say there were more where we did the same thing and a baby was born with no signs of distress), and, sadly, I don't see it getting better anytime soon. But before I get too negative, let me describe what EFM is and how you can ask for it to be used in an evidence-based way in your birth.

Fetal monitoring refers to technology that allows us to trace your baby's heart rate and your uterine activity. This can be done by wearing external monitors that stay on your belly with elastic bands or stickers, or internal monitors that can be placed once your bag of water is broken (more in the next section). This is often done for the entirety of your labor, though there is something called **intermittent monitoring,** which I'll get to in a bit.

The goal of this monitoring is so that we can make sure your baby is doing OK and getting enough oxygen to their brain, which is reflected by their heart rate. You'll often hear us talk about heart rate baseline (the actual heart rate), accelerations (which we love), decelerations (which can be good or bad), variability (how squiggly the heart rate tracing, compared to flat), and how often your contractions are happening.

We take all of this information in and try to interpret whether your baby is getting the oxygen they need and thus they are tolerating labor well, or if they are getting stressed and need to be born more quickly. We also need to interpret it all while keeping in mind that some things like medications can affect how your baby's heart rate looks but might not indicate an actual problem.

The problem with this technology is that studies have shown us there's a lot of variability in how two different obstetric providers might interpret a heart rate tracing and decide how to manage it. This could mean one patient is allowed to labor longer, while the other is told she needs a C-section. Super frustrating, right? And yet here we are.

So with all of this information, here is Dr. Jen's Take on the Technology She Sometimes Can't Stand but Also Can't Ever Stop Using but Hopes We Can Use More Wisely and Not Overact:

1. Consider asking for intermittent monitoring or auscultation. See the box "Intermittent Fetal Monitoring" on the next page).
2. Know that if we're inducing your labor, we will likely need to use continuous monitoring to make sure we are doing it safely. Without it, we might not know if your uterus is contracting too much or if your baby isn't tolerating the medicine we're using.
3. If your team seems worried about your baby's heart rate, ask them to explain why and what things they recommend to make it better (such as stopping Pitocin or having you change positions).
4. If they're recommending internal monitoring, I've got you covered in the next section.
5. If a major intervention like a C-section or forceps or vacuum delivery is recommended because of the tracing and you have concerns, ask to have another obstetric provider review it if there is time (meaning it's not an emergency).
6. Know that for high-risk scenarios (preterm labor, preeclampsia, prior C-section, having an epidural, and more) continuous fetal monitoring is usually recommended because the conditions we're trying to prevent are more likely.
7. If you are really set on no monitoring at all, then a hospital might not be the best place for you. I'm not saying it's not possible, but you might feel more at home in a birth center (or at home).

Intermittent fetal monitoring	
What it is: Using a handheld Doppler device to listen to your baby's heart rate intermittently rather than continuously monitoring it	
Benefits:	• May allow more freedom of movement • May be just as safe as continuous monitoring in low-risk pregnancies
Drawbacks:	• Not all hospitals may be used to doing this and may resist it • Requires 1:1 nurse-to-patient ratio • Optimal protocol for monitoring not established, so your hospital may vary
General recommendations	
Active labor:	Listen every 15–30 minutes
Pushing:	Listen every 5 minutes
Other:	Listen when your bag of water breaks, listen when you are given certain medications, etc.

Head to the Resources section (page 297) for a link to a sample protocol for intermittent fetal monitoring if your team doesn't have one.

AND THEY WANT TO PUT MONITORS . . . INSIDE OF ME?

These are called **internal monitors,** which are placed during a vaginal exam. They can only be used if your bag of water is broken and your cervix is dilated a little.

There are two types:

Fetal scalp electrode (FSE). This is an internal fetal heart rate monitor. It is a very tiny spiral electrode that slides under the skin of your baby's scalp. It is connected to a wire that we connect to the monitor. It is inserted during a cervical exam via a straw-like tube. We attach the FSE to your baby's scalp in a twisting motion, and then remove the straw and our fingers.

Intrauterine pressure catheter (IUPC). This is a flexible tube that is placed vaginally and floats in the amniotic fluid. Just like with the FSE, it is placed using a straw-like tube that is then removed, with the flexible catheter remaining behind. It has a pressure transducer and can measure exactly how strong your contractions are (as opposed to external monitors, which only tell us when and how long your contractions last). We can use an IUPC to calculate Montevideo units (MVUs), which is a measurement that lets us know if contractions are strong enough to expect your cervix to change and labor to progress. MVUs are considered "adequate" if they are calculated to be 200 mm Hg or more over ten minutes.

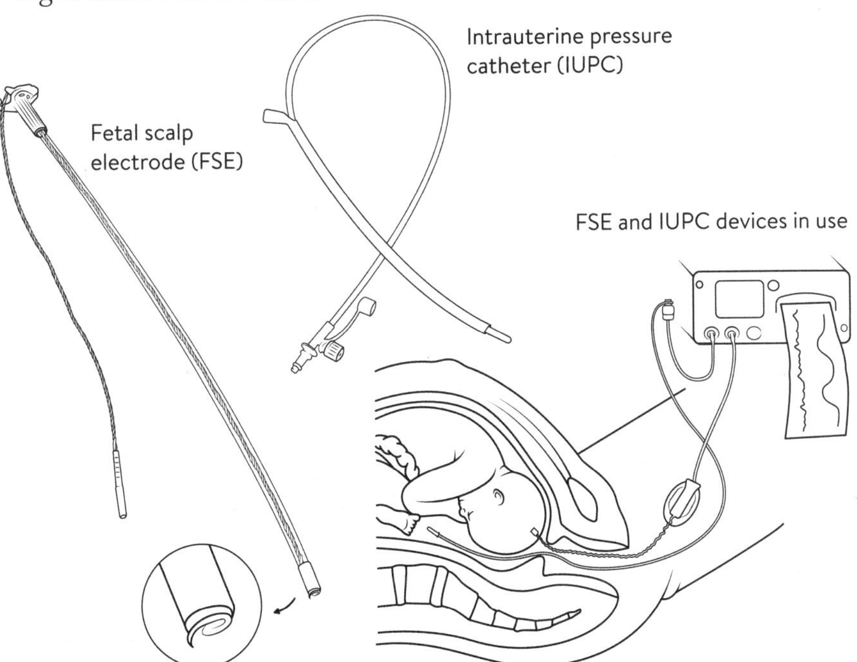

Monitor	Why we use them	Benefits	Risks/concerns	Dr. Jen's notes
Fetal scalp electrode	To more accurately trace your baby's heart rate, since external monitors may not work well because of how your belly is shaped, your baby's movements, the location of your placenta, or if you are frequently changing positions.	· More accurate monitoring. · Allows us to know for certain that we are monitoring your baby's heart rate and not yours. · Less need to readjust external monitors to chase your baby as they move. · Especially helpful if you have twins and we want to be sure we are monitoring two different babies. · Studies do not show an increased risk of infection in labor using this kind of internal monitor. · Use does not increase your C-section risk and may even lower it (since we can see with certainty how your baby is doing).	· There's a 1% risk it leaves a small mark on your baby's head (and a very small risk that this can get infected), but such a mark is often not noticeable or quickly heals. · Requires you to stay connected to the monitor and limits movement. · Concern this might cause your baby pain, though there is no data on this. · Sometimes comes off if your baby has lots of hair, so it may need to be replaced.	These can be especially helpful in an urgent situation where your baby's heart rate has dropped and we are trying to decide if a C-section might be needed but external monitoring isn't adequate. The actual electrode is very tiny, so I don't want that part to scare you off!

Monitor	Why we use them	Benefits	Risks/concerns	Dr. Jen's notes
Intrauterine pressure catheter	• This tells us not only when your contractions are happening but also exactly how strong they are. • We can also do something called an **amnioinfusion** using this, which is where we run IV fluid through the IUPC and into your uterus if we think your baby's umbilical cord is being squished in labor and causing a certain type of heart rate deceleration (variable deceleration).	• Allows us to more accurately know when and how strong contractions are, which can allow us to titrate Pitocin more safely. • If labor is slowing or stalled, this lets us know if the contractions are even strong enough to expect cervical dilation (if not, we can intervene, such as by starting/increasing Pitocin) or, if they are, that a C-section may be warranted.	• Risk of puncturing the placenta or the wall of the uterus during placement. This is not that common and can be minimized by knowing the placental location and stopping if we meet resistance. • About a twofold increased risk of fever. • Can limit your movement.	An IUPC can be crucial in ensuring we don't do a C-section too early, before your contractions are strong enough.

My take-home point on internal monitors is that they are very safe, can help you avoid a C-section in some cases, but are an invasive procedure. **They should *not* be used routinely; they should be reserved for only when we need more information.** If your provider tells you that internal monitors are the "standard protocol" after your bag of water breaks, ask why. I'd be interested in the answer . . .

DO I REALLY NEED AN IV IN MY ARM?

IV stands for "intravenous," and it refers to a catheter that is placed (usually in your forearm) for the purpose of allowing us to give you things like fluids, medicines, and in emergency situations blood transfusions quickly and efficiently.

In general, it is standard to have one in place if you are having a hospital birth. Why? Mainly because we want to stay ahead of the game in case of an emergency, and we need IV access to give medications.

If you are having an induction of labor, want an epidural, or are having a C-section, you'll definitely need an IV. However, if you have a low-risk pregnancy and want to avoid an IV, you have every right to ask about this. In no way can we place one without your consent, and as long as we've reviewed what birthing without an IV might mean and what it could look like if an urgent situation arises, then we've done our part. However, if you know that in the past it's been difficult to have an IV placed, you may want to keep in mind that in an emergency situation this could delay your care. And lastly, if you feel like you're not being heard or respected, see page 137, "What am I allowed to say no to?"

I do often see a misunderstanding of what having an IV means, so here are some myths versus facts to clear things up.

Myth	Fact
Having an IV means I will be hooked up to something.	An IV can be placed and capped off, which means it's there in case you need it, but it's not in use and not hooked up to anything. This is often called a "saline lock" or "hep lock."

Myth	Fact
An IV will restrict my movement.	Even if you have something like fluids running through it, you can still move around. The poles we have it hooked up to are on wheels and can go wherever you go (even in the bathroom). I once had a patient name her IV pole Fred, and wherever she went, Fred went too.
An IV means I will be given medications without my consent.	No! Your consent is always required before we give you anything.
If I have an IV, I can't labor or birth in a tub or shower.	We have waterproof covers we can put on your IV so you can still do these things.
I can wait to get an IV in an emergency.	This is partially true—but you need to know this could delay potentially lifesaving care. Some people have veins that make it hard to get an IV in, and you don't want to discover this in an emergency. It also means that a critical team member like a nurse or anesthesiologist must focus on this rather than doing other things that may be important in a crucial moment.
If I have an IV and they give me fluids, I won't be allowed to eat or drink.	You can still eat and drink with an IV in (more on this in the next section).
IVs hurt!	The placement can, but it's usually very quick. You can also request numbing medicine. It shouldn't hurt once it is in. If it does, let your nurse know so they can make sure it's in correctly or see if it should be moved to a more comfortable spot.
I'll have an IV the whole time I'm in the hospital.	Usually we can remove your IV once you're stable postpartum—often the next day after you've had your baby vaginally, or a day later if you've had a C-section.
I won't be able to hold my baby with an IV.	I promise that you can!
My friend had two IVs and I don't want that.	I hear you—and we only do this if there are high-risk situations like needing a blood transfusion or other very concerning medical issues. This isn't our norm.

CAN I EAT IN LABOR?

My short answer:

- If you're low-risk, it's probably fine to eat what you want.
- If you're at higher risk for a C-section, you probably should stick to lighter food or liquids.
- Hospitals have some pretty outdated policies on this, so don't be surprised if you're told you can only have clear liquids or ice chips once you're in labor or have an epidural—even if you have the lowest-risk of low-risk pregnancies.

So why isn't this so straightforward? Tradition, training, "that's how we've always done it," outdated guidelines, fear of lawsuits, and . . . well, that's really it.

The concern with eating in labor is rooted in the following:

1. Pregnancy slows down your digestive tract, which means food can sit in your stomach longer.

2. The bottom part of your esophagus, which keeps food down, is weaker during pregnancy, which increases your reflux (I probably don't need to tell you this).

3. Pregnancy can make it harder to put a breathing tube in (intubate) because of anatomical changes and swelling in the throat.

4. All of this matters if you need to be put to sleep (especially in an emergency situation) because it can increase your risk of **food aspiration,** which is when food, liquid, and gastric acid come up out of your belly and go into your lungs. This can cause trouble breathing, pneumonia, lung damage, cardiac arrest, and even death.

That sounds scary, right? But just how common is aspiration? Does it happen enough that this "better safe than sorry" attitude around not eating in labor is justified? Here are the numbers, and I'll let you decide:

- Risk of obstetric aspiration in one study: 0.46 percent
- Risk of aspiration during C-sections under general anesthesia in another study: 0.4 percent
- According to one review, this would mean a possible aspiration risk of 1 in every 19,000 births.
- Another study in the United States showed *no* aspirations in over 300,000 births across twenty centers.
- Lastly, one study determined a risk of aspiration at birth leading to cardiac arrest was about 1 in 147,000 births.

Certain risk factors make aspiration risk much higher because of your anatomy or because your stomach empties more slowly, so if any of these apply, you may be advised to not eat in labor, and probably for a valid reason:

- Obesity
- Diabetes
- Using weight-loss drugs (like Ozempic)
- Frequent cannabis use
- Opioid use

These are small numbers, right? Like, *really* small. And we also know that labor is a marathon and has a remarkably high energy requirement, one that IV fluids alone likely can't fulfill. Furthermore, when given the option to eat, laboring people often choose lighter snacks like protein shakes, crackers, or yogurt, not burgers and pizza.

Lastly—and maybe most importantly—**multiple studies have shown being forced not to eat, or not being allowed to eat what you want, causes distress and poor satisfaction after giving birth.**

So, with no data to definitively say that low-risk laboring people can't eat, why do we still see the American College of Obstetricians and Gynecologists and the American Society of Anesthesiologists recommending clear liquids only, while the World Health Organization and many international medical societies call for no or very limited restrictions?

In my opinion, it's because they've got it wrong, and they aren't considering how the mindset of "well, not allowing them to eat can't hurt" is actually *very* distressing to birthing people. When we're forcing our patients to not eat some crackers if they want to and actively ignoring the data that shows how food restriction stresses out many laboring people, it can cause psychological harm, which is far more common than any risk of aspiration.

It is time for us to do better by our patients and leave behind this advice (which originated in the 1940s).

So, what can you do if you're told not to eat or stick to clear liquids? You can:

- Do just that.
- Ask why. If you are told it is hospital policy, ask to see the policy and the references in case you might want to bring this to the attention of your OB-GYN or midwife, or advocate at some point for more updated, evidence-based care at your hospital.
- Let your team know that you are declining that recommendation. They may ask you to sign an against-medical-advice form, which is essentially medico-legal protection for them. If that's the case, you may need to provide your own food and snacks, as they may decline to bring you solid food. In reality, going this route can possibly add friction between you and your care team, and I would be remiss in not mentioning that.

(For my OB-GYN and anesthesia friends who are reading this, I know this might go against how we've been trained. I want you to know that it's OK for us to not always agree with what our patients may choose, but ultimate bodily autonomy means realizing we can still provide amazing care even if we don't see eye to eye. Also: Please read the references for this section and keep an open mind on updating our practices!)

OW! I'M IN PAIN! WHAT CAN I DO?

I'm going to be honest: Labor can be incredibly painful, and anyone who doesn't tell you that is lying. The good news is that we have lots of options to make it better, but some things may not be available at all hospitals—so you know what I'm going to say by now: Ask what your hospital offers long before it's go time, so that you know what's available to you!

Here are some ways to help with labor pain:

1. **Do nothing.** Yes, some people choose to not have anything for pain in labor, and that's totally an OK choice! I did it with my second, and I'll say it was hard but also tolerable because it was what I wanted. I also knew what to expect, so I felt prepared.
2. **Use non-pharmacologic methods.** That is, ways to make pain better without using drugs. There are a *lot* of options here and many birthing people use one or a combo of these. This can include guided breathing, hypnosis, position changes, laboring on a birthing ball, massage, acupuncture or acupressure, or aromatherapy. Below I've highlighted a few other non-drug methods for pain relief in this list that I think deserve some extra discussion.

3. **Have continuous labor support.** This may seem out there, but the evidence shows that having a person or people supporting you in labor decreases the need for pain medications. This could be in the form of a nurse or midwife who is with you continuously, or via the support of a doula, partner, friend, or family member. See page 31, "Do I need a doula?," for lots more on doulas and why they can be an amazing addition to your birth team.

4. **Try hydrotherapy or water immersion.** Data shows that laboring in a tub is associated with less need for pain medications, potentially shorter labors, and high rates of patient satisfaction. If this sounds like something you want available, you should *definitely* ask your OB-GYN or midwife if tubs are available in your hospital (and if they are, are they in every room, or is it first come, first served?) and what the culture is around water immersion for laboring. You can also use the shower in your room if tubs aren't available (pack shower shoes!).

5. **Use a TENS unit.** A transcutaneous electrical nerve stimulation (TENS) device is a tiny unit that sends electrical impulses to little sticky patches you wear. The concept is that the electrical stimulation from the unit blocks or dampens the sensation of pain. Think of it as your brain can only interpret so much info coming from nerves, and the TENS signals drown out some of the painful messages being sent to your brain. These can easily be found in drugstores, and you can keep one in your labor bag if you think you might want to use it. Data shows that for many folks, using a TENS unit decreases the need for pain medication in labor, with really no downside.

6. **Get sterile water injections.** Like it sounds, this is the injection of sterile water under the skin. It is mainly to help with low back pain in labor, often called back labor. We don't quite know why it works, but the theory is that the pain from the injection draws the brain's attention away from the laboring pain, possibly like how a TENS unit works. Sterile water injections are usually a combination of

four injections in the back, and though the injections can hurt while going in, relief happens usually within a matter of minutes and can last a few hours (and they can be repeated). Full disclosure: I have never seen these done (yet!) and this isn't widely practiced in the United States among OB-GYNs, so it's something to bring up with your provider ahead of time to see if they might be comfortable doing this. The evidence shows they work, so I'd love to see this become a more routine practice.

7. **Get an epidural.** This is probably the thing most people think of when they think of pain management in labor, and with good reason, since over 60 percent of people birthing in the United States get one. I go into way more detail about epidurals in the next section, so be sure to check that out if you are considering one.

8. **Have IV pain medication.** These are medications like fentanyl that help ease the pain of contractions but often don't take it away completely. I tell patients it's like having a margarita and caring a little less about your contractions. These can be great options earlier in labor or if you think you might want an epidural but don't want it quite yet. IV pain medication also tends to wear off pretty quickly, so you may need doses repeated every hour or less. We tend to not recommend these right before you birth, as those medications can make your baby a little sleepy and not so excited to breathe on their own, so be aware this probably won't be an option as you are actively birthing your baby.

9. **Use local anesthesia.** This entails us injecting numbing medicine like lidocaine into the nerves that go to the uterus (called a pudendal block), or in the vagina if you've torn during birth and need stitches for a repair. Pudendal blocks aren't done that frequently anymore, but it can definitely be something to try if you're close to delivering, don't have an epidural, and want something.

10. **Use inhaled nitrous oxide.** Yes, kind of like the laughing gas at the dentist! This method of pain control is hardly new and has been

more commonly used in places like the United Kingdom, but it's making a comeback in the United States (and I'm glad it is). What's cool about this method is that it is patient-administered, meaning the laboring person holds the mask or mouthpiece and inhales, and when they've gotten good relief, they remove it. It can be a great option for early labor especially, but even after birth for a laceration repair if someone had no pain relief but needs something for this. Studies have shown it doesn't work as well as an epidural—it's not going to take away your pain completely, though it helps as a coping tool—but it's great to have more options, especially for early labor or for someone who wants to have a bit more freedom of movement than with an epidural.

WHAT IS GETTING AN EPIDURAL LIKE?

If you've seen what an epidural needle looks like on TikTok or elsewhere, you might be freaking out a bit—but I want to reassure you that the placement is often quick and uneventful, and the pain relief that comes after is fantastic!

WHAT TO KNOW WHEN CONSIDERING AN EPIDURAL

Think about these factors so you know when you might want to ask for one:

1. How quickly your anesthesiologist comes depends on if they're in the hospital or dealing with other emergencies.
2. You need to hold still during placement.
3. It can take several minutes to place.
4. It takes ten to twenty minutes to work.

Here's how getting an epidural usually goes:

1. You tell your nurse you want one. They will then call the anesthesia provider and get their ETA.

2. In preparation, you'll usually have some IV fluids given. This is because an epidural can lower your blood pressure. IV fluids counteract too big of a drop, which could make you feel dizzy or nauseated or could drop your baby's heart rate.

3. The anesthesiologist will come in and review the procedure, as well as risks and benefits. You get all your questions answered, and then if you want to proceed you sign on the dotted line. **Pro tip: You can ask for this when you're admitted so that when it's go time for the epidural, you've already done this part when you're not in pain.**

4. Many hospitals will have support folks step out for this procedure and head to the waiting room, but others let them stay. If you're especially nervous and don't want your support person to leave, it never hurts to ask.

5. You will sit up in bed cross-legged or with your legs off the side of the bed (occasionally this can be done with you lying on your side, too). The bed will be raised so that the anesthesiologist can more easily place the epidural in the lower part of your back.

6. They'll push with their fingers to get an idea of your anatomy and figure out where they want to place the needle in the lower part of your back. On occasion, they may use an ultrasound to help identify landmarks. After this, they'll clean off your back with a sterile cleanser and place a sticky drape around the area to keep it tidy.

7. Time to pretend you're a cat! To open up the spaces in your spine, it is most helpful to arch your back like a scared cat or visualize yourself making the letter "C," with your chin touching your chest. Your nurse and anesthesiologist will guide you.

8. Numbing medicine is then injected under the skin and in the space where the epidural needle and catheter will go. You may feel a sensation like an electric shock going down one leg—this is normal and not a cause for concern. Positioning is super important, so your provider may have you make a few minor adjustments throughout—that's normal too.
9. The epidural needle is then placed into your back until it is in the right spot. This can take a single try or a few, depending on your anatomy.
10. Sometimes the anesthesia provider will inject a small amount of medicine into your spinal space while they are placing the epidural. This is called **spinal anesthesia** and allows you to get pain relief quicker as you wait for the epidural to take effect.
11. The catheter (which is a flexible tube that delivers a continuous stream of the numbing medication) is then threaded through the needle, and the needle is taken out. The catheter is secured in place with tape and the plastic drape is removed.
12. A test dose is given to make sure the catheter is in the right place and safe to use.
13. You'll lie back down, and within a few minutes your nurse will check to see if you're starting to feel tingly or numb legs, which confirms it's in the right spot and working.
14. Since you no longer will be able to feel your bladder filling, your nurse may place a catheter to drain your bladder and leave it in place. Another option is using a temporary in-and-out catheter every few hours.
15. Pain relief often happens ten to twenty minutes after placement. Once it kicks in, now is a great time to get a nap!
16. You'll likely see your anesthesia team again at some point as they check in to make sure the epidural is working well. You are free to name your baby after them for all the relief they've given you!

I do want to highlight that **an epidural doesn't stop working after a certain amount of time.** While the catheter can sometimes migrate in longer labors, it's a continuous infusion, and unlike a spinal (which we might use for C-sections), it's not a one-time injection of numbing medicine. You may also have a button you can push for an additional dose if needed. But if it feels like it's no longer working, your nurse and anesthesiologist can troubleshoot to get you better relief, which might include position changes, giving you a "catch-up" dose of medicine by increasing the infusion dose, or replacing the epidural if they think it's moved.

Epidurals come with lots of myths, so let's cover them!

Myth	Fact	Dr. Jen's notes
Epidurals make your labor longer.	On average, people with an epidural push for about fifteen to twenty minutes longer . . .	. . . but you might not mind, since you are more comfortable.
Epidurals increase your chance of needing a forceps or vacuum delivery.	They don't (older data said yes, but more recent studies do not show an increased risk, likely due to us using lower epidural doses).	Check out page 186, "What is the best position to push and deliver my baby in?," if you want to know the best positions to push with an epidural.
Epidurals increase your chance of needing a C-section.	They don't—really!	I hear this one *a lot*, and I tell patients that sometimes an epidural seems to actually allow the pelvic floor to relax, thus *decreasing* the chance of a C-section, but I don't have data to back that up.
Epidurals make it too hard to push effectively.	If you're completely numb, this could be true. But if that's the case, we can turn down the epidural so that you have more sensation to guide your pushing.	

Myth	Fact	Dr. Jen's notes
All epidurals can leave you with areas that still hurt.	This can happen in some, but not most, epidurals. Sometimes we refer to this as a "patchy" epidural or one with a "window" where that area isn't getting pain relief—like a small part of your stomach, for example.	It can suck if one area is not getting the same (or any) relief as other areas. Sometimes position changes or altering the dose can help, and other times we can replace the epidural entirely.
Epidurals cause long-lasting low back pain.	They don't. Back pain after having a baby can be from pushing, pelvic floor weakness, and anatomic changes to your body after giving birth—but we often see the epidural get blamed.	Short-term bruising or soreness may happen, but lifelong back pain and epidurals have never been linked. This is a popular belief in some communities, but we just don't see it when it's studied.
Having an epidural makes it harder to breastfeed.	Studies disagree on this. But with normal epidural doses and being mindful of not overdoing IV fluids (which could lead to breast engorgement), there is likely minimal to no effect on breastfeeding, either for you or for your baby.	If you have concerns, ensuring immediate skin-to-skin contact and asking for lactation help is always a great idea—see page 244, "Who can help me with breastfeeding?"
Epidurals cause autism.	This has not been shown in multiple studies. It also doesn't make sense biologically how an epidural would cause something like autism in a baby.	This concern started after a paper was published in 2020 that showed increased autism rates in the babies of women who had epidurals during labor. Studies since then have shown no linkage, and multiple issues have arisen from the original study. I would *not* be concerned about this.

The following are normal side effects of epidurals we see, and how we deal with them:

Itchy skin	This is not an allergy but a common and normal side effect of the epidural medication. If very bothersome, we can give medications to treat it.
Shivering or “the shakes”	Normal, but can be annoying. The best way to manage is to not try to fight the shakes. If it’s very bothersome, medication can be given to help.
Fever	Can be seen in up to 25% of folks who get an epidural, but this is not a true infection. See page 171, “Why do I have a fever in labor?”
Drop in blood pressure	This happens in about 10% of patients and is caused by a relaxation in your blood vessels. This can be prevented with IV fluids and treated with medications if it occurs. If your blood pressure drops very low, it can also drop your baby’s heart rate, but this often resolves when your blood pressure is treated.
Headaches	Rarely (0.5–1.5% of the time) an epidural can cause a postdural puncture headache (where a tiny amount of spinal fluid leaks). Symptoms include a headache that starts with sitting up but improves with lying down, and usually show up within two days if it’s going to happen. It often heals on its own but can take several days. For quicker relief, the treatment is an **epidural blood patch.** It is another procedure similar to putting in your epidural but can be very effective and can be done before you leave the hospital. If you’re home when these symptoms begin, call us ASAP so we can help!

Unfortunately, there are certain situations where an epidural cannot be safely placed. These include rare genetic diseases, a history of complex back surgery, being on blood thinners, or having a very low platelet count, to name a few. Your team will likely try to create a plan for you ahead of time if you fall into one of these categories, but the good news is that most people who want an epidural can have one!

WHAT IS THE BEST POSITION TO LABOR IN?

The best position is the one that feels right for you and is safe for you and your baby.

But if by "best" you mean the one that will increase your chances of having a successful vaginal birth, let's talk about it.

From a research standpoint **there is no one position that has been found to be the absolute winner.** As you can imagine, this is hard to study in a high-quality way! The average laboring person will spend time in many different positions, such as lying down, bouncing on a birthing ball, walking the halls, and so on.

Still, I will share with you some data that we *do* have, with a big caveat that some of it isn't the best quality, but it's what we've got:

Effect on . . .	Being upright (i.e., walking, sitting on a birthing ball, or kneeling)	Water immersion* (laboring in a tub)
First stage of labor	Shortened by over an hour	Shortened by thirty minutes
Having an epidural	Decreased rates of having an epidural	
Chance of needing a C-section	Decreased by 30%	No difference
Any harm to the pregnant patient or their baby	Not associated with any harm	

Note: This refers only to laboring in a tub, not to actually giving birth in one. For more on that, head to page 23, "Should I have a waterbirth?"

These kind of make sense, right? Being upright helps gravity do its thing and move your baby down in the pelvis, and theoretically it can encourage your baby's head to be in an optimal position for the grand exit. And being in a relaxing tub of warm water can help relieve labor pain.

However, I *do* want to stress that you are not harming yourself or your baby if you choose to lie down, get an epidural, or get out of the tub. **Your decision to rest in bed is not to blame if you end up needing a C-section.**

Remember, these studies weren't all great, and many things can factor into needing a C-section. If I sound like I'm belaboring (ha) this point, it's because I can see what guilt does to a birth story, and I do not want this for you.

My takeaways on this are:

1. If you're in labor, you should be informed of the benefits of being upright (based on limited data) or in the water.
2. You can be upright with an epidural, but it takes some positioning to make it safer so you don't fall.
3. Unless there is a medical concern where being in bed is recommended (and yes, those do exist), then you should be free to labor and be supported in whatever position feels good for you.
4. Your body knows best what it needs.

HOW OFTEN WILL THEY CHECK MY CERVIX?

There should be no routine number of cervical exams when you're in labor. If an OB-GYN is reading this and disagrees with me because you were trained to do cervical exams every two hours (or at other intervals) like I was, I'm going to politely/desperately ask you to change your practice.

Why? Because cervical exams should only be done when they are needed, such as if it would change our management or if we have concerns. These exams, which involve us using two fingers to see how opened and shortened the cervix is and where the position of the baby's head is, are not totally benign. They can be uncomfortable and feel intrusive, and they can increase the risk of infection if someone's bag of water is broken.

So that's why I can't really say how often your cervix might be checked, other than to say it's well within your right to ask why it's being recommended and what decision point it is needed for. If there's not a great answer and you're not feeling it, you can decline it or ask for some more time before you're checked. Yes, there are times where we really need to know. In those scenarios your team should make this clear, and when this happens with my patients I try to communicate this urgency but again respect their autonomy.

Bonus tip: Ask this question of your doctor or midwife at a prenatal visit to see where their practice lies. This can help you feel out whether this team feels right for you and reassure you that you've had this conversation long before labor has even begun!

I WAS TOLD I'M GBS POSITIVE AND I'M FREAKING OUT.

Please don't freak out! This is super common, and I don't want you to panic.

GBS stands for **group B streptococcus,** which is an entirely normal bacteria that up to 30 percent of us carry in our bodies. It does not cause us any harm, but it *can* be an issue for babies when they pass through the birth canal if they're exposed to it. Babies exposed to GBS can get very sick with pneumonia, sepsis (infection in their bloodstream that also affects their organs), and brain infections. Before we screened all pregnant people, this used to be the most common reason newborn babies went to the neonatal intensive care unit.

Enter universal screening: We now test everyone who is pregnant for GBS so that if they do carry it, we can treat them in labor to decrease the chance that their baby will be exposed. The test is done with a quick swab in the vagina and rectum (both places where GBS can live), usually between 36 and 38 weeks of pregnancy. Sometimes we test earlier if we think you might deliver preterm. If GBS is detected in a urine culture at some point in your pregnancy, that also "counts" as having GBS (even if you've been treated), as does having a baby who got sick from GBS before.

If you carry GBS, the treatment is super easy. We just give IV antibiotics while you're in labor (and not continuously, so you aren't hooked up to an IV during your entire labor). The usual treatment is penicillin, but if you have an allergy, we can use something else. While this doesn't completely eliminate the threat GBS poses to your baby, it does decrease it to only about 0.25 percent.

But what about . . .	
Why not give me antibiotics when I'm pregnant to protect my baby from it?	The actual risk from GBS is exposure as your baby passes through the birth canal and especially after your water is broken. No need for treatment in pregnancy!
Can I take antibiotics or something natural when I'm pregnant to try to clear it before I go into labor?	I've seen some practitioners recommend probiotics, placing garlic in the vagina, colloidal silver, dietary changes, or certain supplements to clear up GBS before you give birth. Studies either never have been done or do not show enough of a benefit to replace using antibiotics. And some of these practices can cause harm—not all that is natural is risk-free.
Since I'll need IV antibiotics, does this mean I can't have a homebirth or birth center birth?	Not necessarily! Some midwives can administer IV antibiotics in your home or a birth center, which means you can get the treatment you need without having to have a hospital birth. See page 20, "I'm going the homebirth/birth center route—what now?"

But what about . . .	
Can I decline testing or treatment?	You can always choose what to do, but I'd think this one through. If you're GBS positive, you have a 50% chance your baby will get GBS from you, and a 1–2% chance they will get very sick or die (which goes up to 19% if they are preterm). The overall risk is low, but it's real. GBS is not an infection to mess around with in a new baby; however, the choice is ultimately yours.
Is GBS a sexually transmitted infection?	No.
If I had it in one pregnancy, will I always have it?	Nope—it can come and go, which is why we test in every pregnancy.
Do I need to be tested if I'm planning a C-section?	We do recommend it in case you change your mind or birth vaginally before we're able to perform your C-section. It also helps the pediatricians if your baby gets sick in the first month of life and they want to identify any possible exposures.
Do I need to be treated if I'm having a C-section?	No, because the antibiotics we give to prevent C-section infections actually cover GBS, so there's no need for a separate medication.
If I had GBS in my urine and take antibiotics, will it clear it just like any other urinary tract infection?	Unfortunately, no. If you have it in your urine, it's assumed that you carry a very high amount of GBS in your genital area. This means we highly recommend IV antibiotics in labor—even if you took oral antibiotics to treat a UTI in your pregnancy.

MY DOCTOR WANTS TO BREAK MY BAG OF WATER AND I'M NOT SURE IF I SHOULD.

Amniotomy is the technical term for when we break the bag of waters. We use a tiny sterile hook either at the end of something that looks like a crochet needle or worn on the finger to do this.

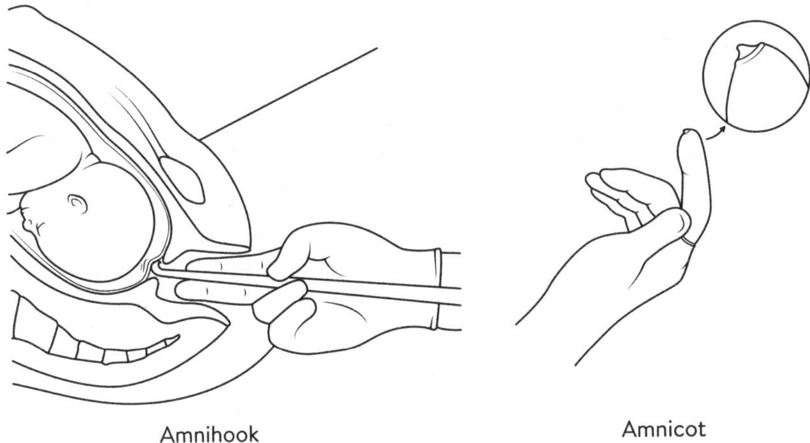

The idea is that the breaking of the bag of water helps your baby's head press down on the cervix more, thereby helping it dilate. It can also cause the release of chemical messengers called prostaglandins, which can make your contractions stronger and more frequent—and yes, oftentimes more painful.

If your doctor or midwife suggests breaking your bag of water rather than waiting for it to happen on its own, here's what you can ask:

1. For what benefit are you suggesting this?
2. Are there any risks?
3. Is this urgent or an emergency, or can we have some time to think about it?

If your provider answers with "We routinely do this for all patients," I want to highlight that **the routine breaking of the bag of waters shouldn't be a thing.** Studies show us there's no benefit to routinely using this intervention in someone in spontaneous labor, and it doesn't shorten labor or increase your chances of a vaginal birth.

However, it *can* have a role in some scenarios:

1. **Internal monitoring.** If we are unable to monitor your baby or your contractions using external monitors (see page 98, "And they want to put monitors . . . inside of me?"), there is an option to use internal monitors but—you guessed it—your bag of water must be broken for us to be able to do this.

2. **Helping labor along.** If you're undergoing a labor induction, or if your labor has slowed and your team suggests interventions to help you progress (see pages 80, "How does an induction work?," and 127, "They say my labor is going too slowly—what does that mean?"), breaking your bag often in conjunction with IV oxytocin has been shown to shorten the length of labor and decrease the need for a C-section.

Risks include:

1. **Umbilical cord prolapse.** This is when the cord comes down into the vagina, often leading to an urgent C-section. This is very rare (about 0.2 percent risk). Ask your provider if your baby's head is low enough in the pelvis to decrease the chances of this happening before they break your bag of water.

2. **Abnormal fetal heart rate tracing.** Now that the cushion of fluid is gone, sometimes the cord can get squished and drop the baby's heart rate. Luckily, this is often treatable by changing your position or using something called an amnioinfusion, which is described on page 98, "And they want to put monitors . . . inside of me?"

3. **Increased risk of infection.** If you have a long labor after the bag of water is broken or undergo many cervical exams, your risk of

infection increases. This is because the protective barrier of the bag of water is no longer there, and bacteria can get into the uterus more easily.

Like many things related to labor and birth, having your bag of water broken is not always good nor always harmful and can often be helpful, so I hope this information helps you make an informed decision with your obstetric team.

SHOULD I BE WORRIED ABOUT MECONIUM IN MY AMNIOTIC FLUID?

Meconium is your baby's first poop, and you usually see it within the first day or two after birth. It's that sticky stuff that can be *really* hard to wipe off. However, about 10 to 20 percent of babies (and even higher in those past their due date) will have their first bowel movement when they're still in the uterus. This leads to meconium-stained amniotic fluid.

When we see meconium-stained amniotic fluid, we note it and pay attention because it can indicate that your baby is or was feeling a little stressed, and that's why they pooped. But it's not a guarantee that there was anything wrong or that there will be.

Meconium, when breathed in either in the uterus or at the time of birth, can cause inflammation and blockages in a baby's lungs. This can lead to **meconium aspiration syndrome**. Babies with this have trouble breathing, abnormally low oxygen levels, and low heart rates. They may need NICU admission and extra breathing help through intubation.

I know that sounds scary! But I want you to know the actual numbers, which can help reassure you:

- Eighty to 90 percent of these babies will be born crying and breathing just fine. Nothing different will need to be done to care for them when they arrive.
- Meconium aspiration syndrome happens in only 1 to 5 percent of babies with meconium-stained fluid, with those higher numbers in those who are post-term or have had an abnormal fetal heart rate tracing while in labor.

If your baby has meconium-stained fluid, we will likely:

1. Recommend continuous fetal monitoring to keep an eye out for any signs of distress.
2. Consider having a neonatal resuscitation team member at your birth (though this isn't done everywhere, such as my hospital, where we have nurses who can start any needed breathing help and then call the NICU team if needed).

If you have meconium and you are worried, ask your team if *they* are worried, and what they're doing to monitor your baby to ensure a safe arrival.

WHAT IS PITOCIN AND WHY MIGHT THEY SUGGEST I NEED IT?

Oxytocin is a hormone your body makes that is responsible for uterine contractions. Pitocin is the synthetic version of this, and we can give it intravenously to help speed up or induce your labor and to help prevent or treat heavy bleeding.

Pitocin is used in about 30 percent of all people who give birth vaginally in a hospital in the United States. There's a good chance you might hear about it, so let's review! But before I do, I want to stress that **there is no place for routine Pitocin to be used on every patient to speed up labor**—it should only be used when there is a reason that we think it may help.

Pitocin given in your IV is not a set dose. The rate of flow can be increased up or down with the goal of getting your uterus to contract every few minutes, with enough time for you and your baby to get a break between contractions. We usually see an effect about thirty minutes after we start the infusion. Sometimes we start Pitocin to get you into more active labor, and then once that happens it can be turned off as your body's own oxytocin takes over.

For labor induction

See page 80, "How does an induction work?," for more on how labor is induced and when Pitocin would be used (and when it shouldn't).

For a slow or stalled labor

Pitocin can be used to speed up both latent and active labor (for a refresher on these terms, see page 93, "What is normal labor, anyway?"). If your cervix has stopped dilating, using Pitocin (often in combination with breaking your bag of water) and giving it time to work should be tried if possible before jumping to a C-section, as this has been shown to increase vaginal birth rates. I've got more on this in the next section as well.

For the prevention of bleeding

Pitocin given after your baby is born helps your uterus contract to prevent excessive postpartum bleeding. This is often recommended for all patients (my exception to the no-Pitocin-for-everyone rule!), as we know it is the most effective medication to prevent postpartum hemorrhage, which can be a life-threatening complication of childbirth. In this scenario, it can be given through your IV or as a shot in your thigh.

For the treatment of heavy bleeding

Pitocin is often the go-to medicine used to stop heavy bleeding after a vaginal birth or C-section. Other medicines can also be used, but this is often our first-line treatment, as it works so well and has the least side effects.

There are some risks to Pitocin use that you should be aware of:

1. **Causing too many uterine contractions.** This can stress your baby out and lead to fetal heart rate changes that reflect that. This can be fixed by stopping or decreasing the Pitocin, or giving a medication called **terbutaline,** which counteracts it.

2. **Pain.** I often get asked if Pitocin contractions hurt worse than your own natural ones, and my response is always that labor contractions hurt regardless of why they're happening. It's not that Pitocin causes super-strength contractions—it's just that it's working and your body is contracting effectively; before we started the Pitocin, that may not have been the case, which is why it didn't feel as intense.

3. **The need to be monitored.** We need to monitor your baby's heart rate and contractions continuously if you're on Pitocin so that we can ensure we're using the right dose. Because of this, intermittent monitoring, which I discuss on page 95, "Talk to me about fetal monitoring," isn't recommended here.

4. **Uterine rupture.** This is rare, thankfully, but there's a higher risk if you've had a C-section before. More on this on page 33, "Can I just request a C-section?"

If your provider is recommending Pitocin, ask why so that you understand the rationale. You can always decline, ask for more time, or ask for alternatives. Just know that in emergency scenarios like a hemorrhage, we may be pressed for time and even if you thought you'd never want Pitocin as part of your birth plan, this might be a time to consider an exception.

THEY SAY MY LABOR IS GOING TOO SLOWLY—WHAT DOES THAT MEAN?

Let's talk about it! Head back to page 93, "What is normal labor, anyway?," to review the stages of labor and what we consider "normal" for each stage. If your provider says that your labor is progressing slower than expected, they mean that the rate at which your cervix is opening and thinning out is slower than what they would expect in a typical labor, or that your baby isn't coming down in the birth canal in the usual way we see.

I'm going to confess something here: My field can be known for not giving labor enough time and for too quickly labeling someone's labor as "too slow" or "abnormal." This can lead to increased interventions like use of Pitocin, breaking your bag of water, placing internal monitors, and performing C-sections more often than we need to.

That said, labor can absolutely be protracted, or slower, than is considered physiologically normal. And this can lead to increased risks of infection, bleeding, need for C-section, and stress or infection in your baby that may result in their admission to the NICU.

So, it's important to tease out what is truly too slow from what just may be a bit of impatience.

I'm hoping this table and flow chart can help if this happens in your labor and you'd like some guidance on how to approach these conversations:

		What we may recommend	Dr. Jen's notes
Stage 1			
Prolonged labor	Cervical change that is happening, but slower than expected. This can be less than 0.5–1 cm an hour.	· Patience! · Position changes (being upright) · Breaking the bag of water · Pitocin	If you're in latent labor or being induced, this can be hours to days and still be normal, so it's important not to move to a C-section too quickly in this situation.
Arrest of active labor (at least 6 cm dilated, with bag of water broken)	No cervical change after four hours (if adequate contractions) or six hours (if inadequate contractions)	· Position changes · Pitocin	We measure if contractions are "adequate" using an intrauterine pressure catheter (IUPC)—see page 95, "Talk to me about fetal monitoring."
Stage 2			
Prolonged	Still pushing after two hours (if you've had a vaginal birth before) or three hours (if it's your first time)	· Position changes · Pitocin · Forceps or vacuum delivery · C-section	· We may diagnose this much earlier if when pushing there is absolutely no progress, because this is a sign the baby likely won't fit out and it increases risks to you. · As long as there is some progress, though, it can often be fine to push longer than the times listed here.

Unfortunately, it's not always straightforward. This highlights both the art and science of medicine and having a baby. Having a team you trust can really make the difference here: You know you tried all the things to get your baby out vaginally, and so if a C-section is recommended, you'll know that it truly is best for you and baby.

TALK TO ME ABOUT C-SECTIONS.

WHY WORDS MATTER

I remember being an OB-GYN resident and standing outside a postpartum patient's room one day. I was presenting her case to my team before we would all go in the room to see her.

"Ms. X is post-op day one from a crash C-section—"

"A what?" interrupted my attending, who was one of my favorites in that she loved teaching us . . . but who also was known for her high expectations.

"A crash C-section. I got the baby out in less than a minute and—"

"Would you want to hear that the birth of your baby was a 'crash' event, Dr. Lincoln?" she gently but pointedly suggested.

"Um . . . no?" I replied, while I thought, *Is it not enough that I saved this baby's life? Now I need to worry about* how *I say it?*

"Let's say 'emergent' instead, shall we?" suggested my attending.

"OK. She is post-op day one from an emergent C-section . . ."

Guess what? She was totally right. Words matter, even if in my exhausted state I didn't realize it. I've only come to understand this the longer I practice and the more time I spend on social media hearing from people who felt that words used in their care hurt them or dehumanized their experience.

So thank you, Dr. O'Reilly, for all you've taught me . . . and many other learners!

About one in three births in America happen this way, so knowing what a C-section looks like (even if you really wish to avoid one) isn't a bad idea in terms of being fully informed.

C-sections come in a few flavors:

- **Scheduled/planned.** Like it sounds—these are scheduled in advance and are done before labor begins. This might be if your baby is breech, or you've had a C-section before and make a plan to have another (called a repeat C-section).
- **Unscheduled/unplanned.** This might be that you were in labor and a C-section was deemed necessary, or you had a C-section on the books but your team performed it sooner because you went into labor before your scheduled date.
- **Emergent.** This is a type of unscheduled C-section where either you or your baby is in danger and your team needs to move very quickly. Sometimes called a "crash" C-section (which is a terrible term, as you see me discuss in my story at the start of this section), it can happen within a matter of minutes and, as such, can feel chaotic. You may need to be put to sleep for it if there isn't time for an epidural or spinal anesthetic to be used.

Knowing what to expect can be half the battle. Here's your C-section road map, with the disclaimer that some variation can be normal:

1. **You are told you need a C-section.** See page 190, "They're telling me I need a C-section but I don't think I need one. Can I say no?," for reasons you might need one. You'll have time for a discussion of why this is recommended, an explanation of the process, and a chance to review the risks/benefits/alternatives, and you will sign a surgical consent form.

2. **Your nurse will prepare all the things.** If you come in for a scheduled C-section, you'll have the usual admitting things done (see

page 86, "What happens when I get admitted?"). If you've been in labor, your same labor nurse will help get you ready for your C-section by making sure your IV is working well, possibly drawing blood for certain labs, running IV fluids to prepare your body for anesthesia, and maybe clipping any pubic hair in your bikini line where the incision will be. They will also give you medicine to drink that neutralizes your stomach acid in case you get nauseated and vomit in the operating room. They'll also start IV antibiotics to decrease your risk of infection.

3. **An anesthesiologist will come talk to you.** They will explain the process of placing numbing medicine in your back to take away pain during the C-section but allow you to be awake—this is done either via a spinal block or by dosing up your epidural that you may already have in place for labor. In general, we want to avoid putting you to sleep because being awake means you get to see your baby, placing a breathing tube (intubation) while pregnant is slightly riskier and can leave you with a nasty sore throat, it increases your risk of bleeding, and it also make your baby sleepy and they may need extra breathing support once born. More discussion, more consent forms. They'll also likely give you medicine for nausea in your IV to prevent nausea during the procedure.

WHAT'S THE DIFFERENCE BETWEEN A SPINAL AND AN EPIDURAL?

Both can be used to numb you from the waist down for a C-section. An **epidural** is an indwelling continuous catheter that can be used for pain relief in labor and dosed up for a C-section. A **spinal** is a one-time shot of medicine in your back that lasts for a few hours. We usually use a spinal if you're having a scheduled C-section or didn't have an epidural in labor.

4. **You will go to the operating room (OR).** You and usually one support person will go to the room where your baby will be born! You'll get a cute little bouffant to wear to cover your hair, and your support person will be given a sterile gown to wear over their clothes. Your support person usually waits outside the OR until just before the C-section begins to allow the team to focus just on you while getting set up.

5. **You'll move from your bed to the OR bed.** If you have an epidural, your team will help you shimmy to where you need to be. It can be chilly in the operating room, so we usually have plenty of warm blankets to give you, but speak up if you're still too cold.

6. **Spinal anesthesia is placed.** If you don't have an epidural, then you'll sit upright on the OR table, curl your back like a cat, and have an injection of numbing medicine placed in your back. Your nurse and anesthesiologist will help you get positioned and explain everything that is happening to you. After this you'll lie down and then . . .

7. **Time to feel like the pit crew is at work.** This moment may feel chaotic for even a planned C-section—it's when your nurses, anesthesiologist, OB-GYN, and other helpers do all the things to make sure your birth is as safe as possible: placing EKG leads, monitors, blood pressure cuff, squeezy boots on your legs to prevent blood clots, a bladder catheter to drain your urine (only after you're numb!), a belt so you stay on the OR bed; making sure the baby equipment and surgical tools are all working; and more.

8. **Your abdomen is cleaned.** A nurse will use a sterile solution to clean off your belly and the top of your thighs. This decreases the chance of a surgical infection. Depending on what they use, it can leave your skin blue or pink for a few days after, so don't be scared if you see that! It usually has to dry for a few minutes before . . .

9. **Sterile drapes are placed.** A sterile drape that acts as a divider between you and where your surgeons are working is placed on

your belly. These often have clear windows so that you can see your baby once they are born (or sooner if you want to watch more!).

10. **Anesthesia is double-checked.** Your OB-GYN will pinch your belly with a surgical tool to make sure you don't feel any pain. A sense of pressure and light touch are normal—but pain is not, so tell us if you feel something like a pinch or poke. If you do feel pain, we can wait longer for your anesthesia to take effect, give you medicine in your IV, or, as a last resort, put you to sleep.

11. **Final safety check.** We do something called a "surgical time-out" where everyone in the room pauses and confirms everything is done correctly. The consent form is checked, and we confirm that your antibiotics were given, that all devices are on and functioning, that everyone who needs to be in the room is present, and that any concerns are addressed.

12. **Enter your support person.** After this safety check, your support person is brought in. They usually sit in a chair positioned right next to your head so they can be right by you the entire time.

13. **The C-section begins.** The time from the first incision on your belly to meeting your baby is usually just a few minutes, but it can be longer if there's scar tissue that slows us down. We usually delay cord clamping for about a minute (more about this on page 209, "Should I ask for delayed cord clamping?"), during which time we can show you your baby through the clear drapes. Then, after the cord is cut, your baby often gets taken to the baby warmer, where they are checked out (support folks can come over and snap pictures), and then they're brought over to you for skin-to-skin contact. During this time, your surgeons continue the C-section by delivering your placenta and then stitching up the layers that were entered on the way in. This takes a bit longer, but can average about twenty to thirty minutes.

14. **Time to clean up.** Once your abdominal incision is closed and a bandage is placed, your team will remove the surgical drape. Before they help you shimmy back over to your labor bed, they will do something called a uterine massage where they press down on the top of your uterus to help remove any large clots. Usually you won't feel pain thanks to your anesthesia, but it's normal to feel lots of pressure.

15. **You head out to a recovery room or your previous labor room.** The first few hours after a C-section are a time where you are watched closely—it's a major abdominal surgery, and so we want to keep a close eye on you. Your nurse will be by your side checking your blood pressure frequently, making sure there are no signs of bleeding, ensuring your pain and nausea are under good control, and helping you snuggle with your baby and assist with baby's first feed. Usually visitors (other than your core support team) are asked to wait elsewhere so you can have this special bonding time and allow for closer monitoring.

STAPLES OR STITCHES?

Ask your doctor how they plan to close your incision. We have data to show that stitches under the skin have lower rates of wound complications, so this is usually preferred in most cases over staples.

An emergency C-section is quite different—all the above happens but much more quickly. You may need to be put to sleep, and in that case your support person is not in the operating room. You will wake up feeling groggy and a bit out of it, but our goal is always to get you with your baby ASAP. If you plan to breastfeed, you can do so as soon as you feel awake enough to hold your baby.

Here's a list of some questions you might want to ask at a prenatal visit about how your provider and hospital do C-sections. Even if you aren't planning to have one, this can help you feel prepared if it does happen:

1. Can my support person be in the operating room with me?
2. Is it OK to take pictures and videos?
3. Will you use a clear drape so I can see my baby once they're born?
4. Can you confirm my baby won't leave the operating room unless there is an issue?
5. Am I able to do skin-to-skin in the OR?
6. Is it still routine to do delayed cord clamping unless there is a medical concern?

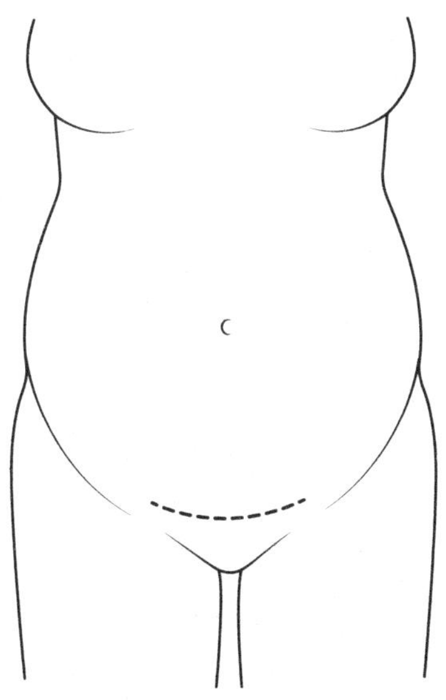

1. The incision is usually just above your bikini line.

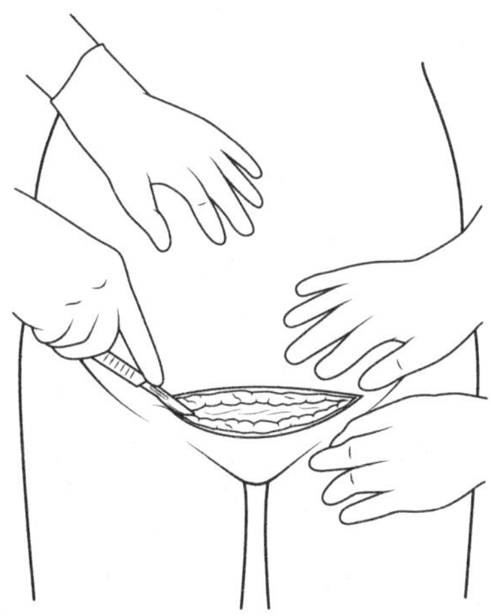

2. A scalpel is used to make the incision through the skin and underlying tissue.

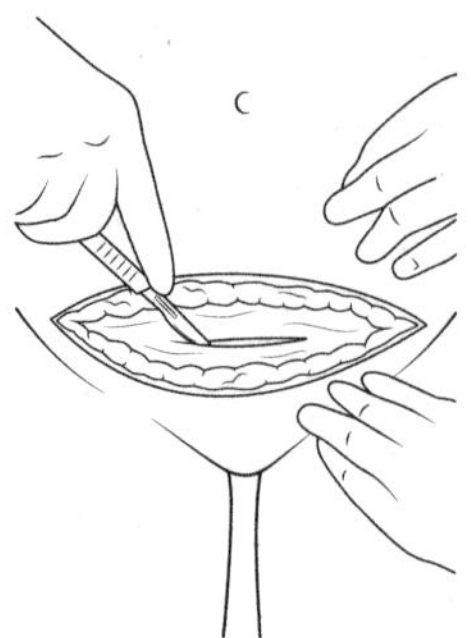

3. The tough tissue that keeps your organs inside, called the fascia, is cut.

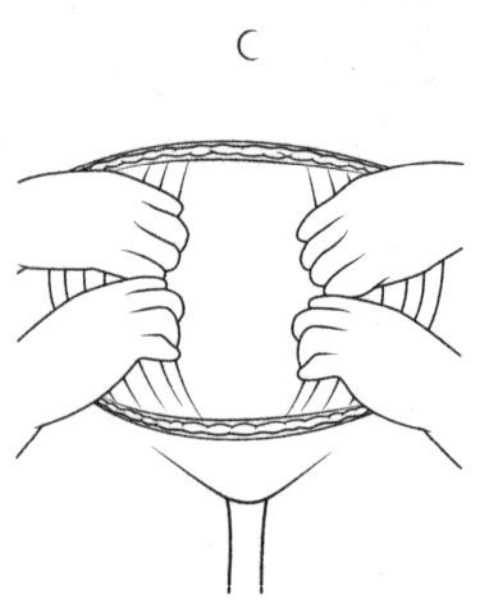

4. Your abdominal muscles are separated to the side.

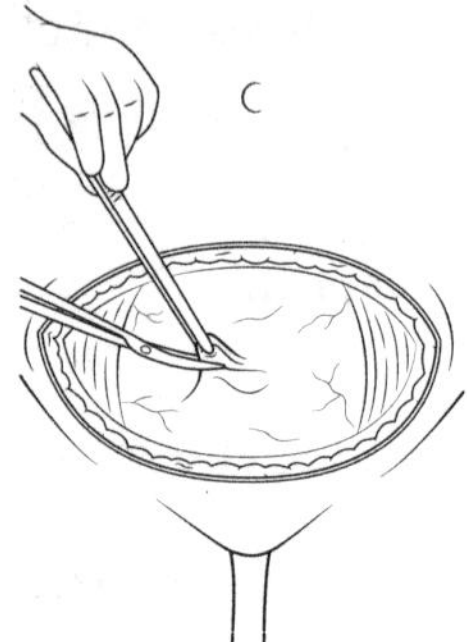

5. We enter the peritoneum, which is a thin membrane that lines your abdomen.

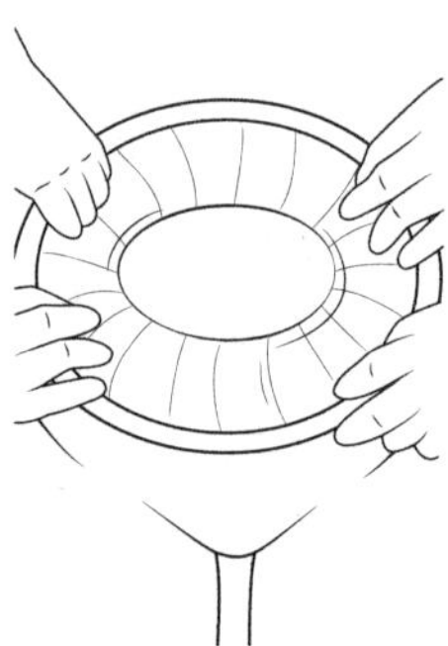

6. An internal retractor may be placed to help us see better.

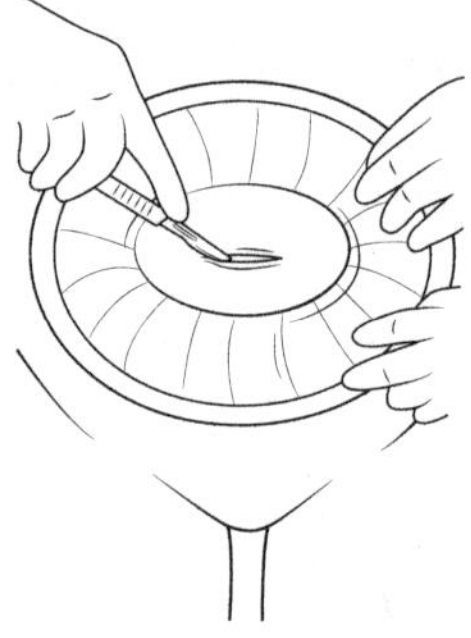

7. An incision is made to open the uterus.

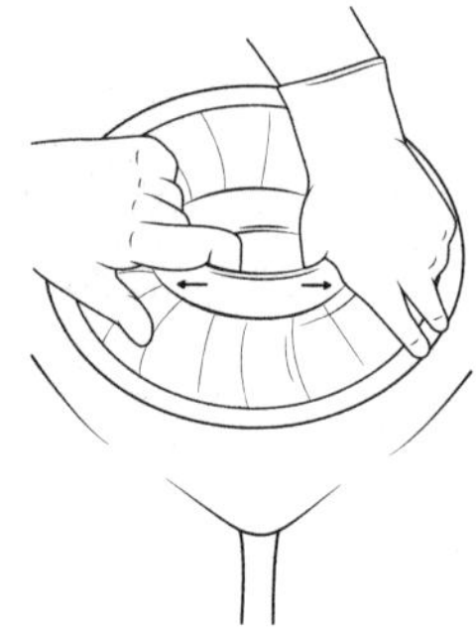

8. We use our fingers to gently extend this incision so your baby will fit out.

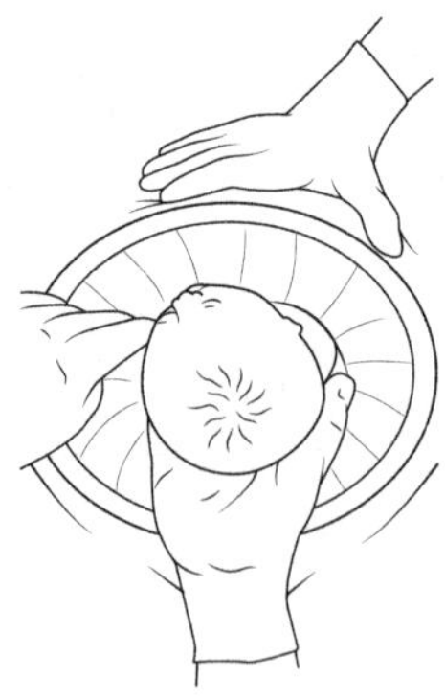

9. We insert our hand to deliver your baby. Our assistant will press on your uterus from above to help with delivery.

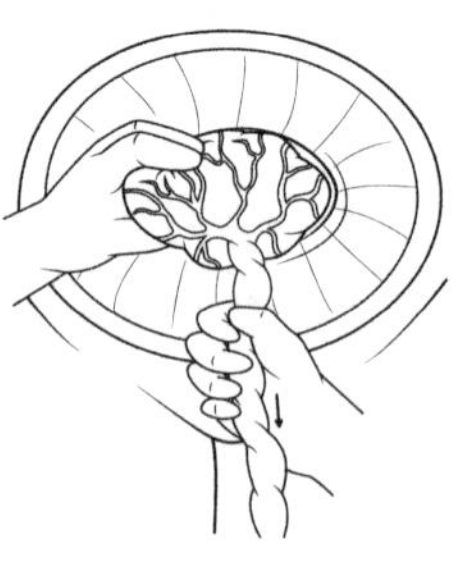

10. After your baby is handed to a nurse, we will guide the placenta out.

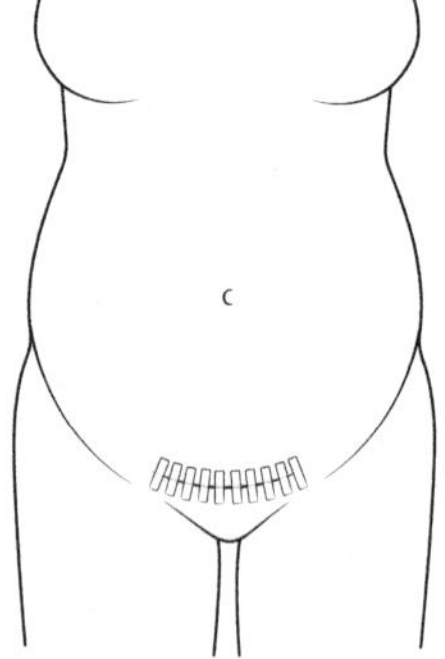

11. We then stitch up the layers we entered and close the skin with stitches (usually).

WHAT AM I ALLOWED TO SAY NO TO?

Basically, anything. This is your body, your labor, your baby—your autonomy is a guiding principle at the end of the day.

I'm not just coming at this from a pro-choice angle, one that I believe in wholeheartedly. It's also a legal matter: We can't legally do anything to you without your consent.

You can say no to staying in the hospital, having an IV, having your blood drawn, fetal monitoring, us checking your vital signs, undergoing a surgery like a C-section, what medications we give you and your baby, and more.

It is our job to explain the risks, benefits, and alternatives of anything we do or recommend. If you choose to decline something and we've had an informed conversation, then I've done my part.

There are definitely times when a choice can harm you or your baby, and it is up to us as your medical team to communicate that. It's also on us to not use fear tactics or blow things out of proportion to coerce you into something we deem routine or no big deal—we need to save the "your baby could die" line for when that could *actually* be true.

There's a balance here, and I strive every day to be clear about when I think a choice my patient makes probably isn't going to cause a problem versus when it could lead to a huge complication. And even in the latter situation, it's ultimately not my choice to make.

Some OB-GYNs will read this and say, "Easy for her to say, but the reality is we can get sued if a patient chooses something and there's a bad outcome, so we have to act this way." They're not wrong about the risk of a lawsuit, but unfortunately this is an ever-present risk in medicine and our field in general. The best defense is not to scare patients or practice defensive medicine but rather to form relationships with our patients, document well, and—if a provider feels they are really being compromised—to transfer care to a different provider if the original one no longer feels comfortable.

We also must own that our field is steeped in a history where women were dismissed, experimented on, and abused. Sometimes not being listened to can cause more trauma to someone in labor than any C-section complication ever could.

The last thing I'll say is I get that it is very different for an upper-class white woman in her thirties to decline a treatment than it is for a single Black nineteen-year-old. There is the real fear of being labeled "difficult" and that Child Protective Services might get called and your baby taken from you if you're the second patient. This isn't hypothetical—data shows Black women are reported more often and their babies removed from them much more than other racial groups.

I keep going back to this, but this is why I think a birth plan/preferences discussed *during* your pregnancy can be so helpful, so that when you show up in labor you and your team know where everyone stands. Let's work on building trust through communication and mutual respect.

I DON'T FEEL I'M BEING LISTENED TO. WHAT ARE MY OPTIONS?

I'm sorry if you're experiencing this. There's nothing more frustrating than feeling that you aren't heard during a process that takes all your mental and physical energy.

I mentioned a bit about going up the chain on page 56, "Should I rush to the hospital if my bag of water broke but I'm not having contractions?," but here are some tactics specifically for when you are in labor:

What you can do	You can say . . .	Dr. Jen's notes
Speak up directly to your nurse or obstetric provider	• "I feel like I'm not being heard. Can we try again?" • "I don't understand why we are doing ___. Can you please explain?"	Sometimes we need the reminder that what's routine to us might not be to you—so this technique might be all you need to get us and your experience back on track.
Have a team member speak up on your behalf	• To your nurse: "I don't feel like Dr. X is giving me enough time to dilate. Can you help me out?" • To your midwife: "My nurse doesn't seem comfortable with me being upright, but this really matters to me—can you figure out what we can do?"	This can help if you don't feel comfortable asking the person directly (for people who may feel targeted for speaking up and being labeled as "difficult," this can be a real, albeit unfair and enraging, concern).
Let your supporters speak up	• Your doula: "We are concerned that the anesthesiologist isn't addressing that the epidural isn't working well, and we'd like someone else to help out." • Your partner: "My girlfriend does best with more information, so please explain ___ again."	If you have a doula, this is absolutely in their job description—which is why having one can be so awesome! But if you don't have one, friends or family members can also be your voice if needed.
Ask to go up the chain	You can ask to speak to the following people who are present in most hospitals: • Charge nurse • Nursing supervisor • Patient advocate	This might feel uncomfortable, but ensuring patient safety—which includes being heard—is part of these job descriptions. Use these folks if needed.
Ask for new team members	• "I don't feel that my nurse and I are clicking. Can I please have a new nurse?" • "My OB-GYN is not listening to me and it's really making this process too hard. Am I able to have a different doctor assigned to me?"	Birth is more intimate than a first date, and like first dates, not all matches work out. Sometimes a switch is possible and sometimes it isn't (if another OB-GYN isn't available, for example), but it doesn't hurt to ask.

Hopefully, you're reading this to be prepared and you never need to utilize any of these tactics. But if you do, remember that clear communication is essential and feeling respected is a human right you are entitled to.

If your birth didn't turn out as you hoped, I do cover birth trauma on page 272, "I think I had a traumatic birth and I don't know where to go for help." You deserve to get the care and support you need.

IF THINGS
GET INTERESTING

OUT OF CHAOS . . .

My patient, Vanessa, had just birthed the head of her baby. She was screaming and saying lots of four-letter words—yes, she was doing this unmedicated.

"I need you to stop pushing. Your baby's shoulder is stuck," I said above her shrieks while her husband was taking photos of said stuck head.

"Get this baby out of me! I can't stop pushing!"

"I really need you to stop. We have a shoulder dystocia," I tried to say in my calmest voice amid the chaos.

I could feel the sweat starting to pool in my armpits. I locked eyes with the nurse, who immediately knew this was my "Oh shit" face, and she called for extra help. She then got up on a stool, flexed my patient's legs back, and pushed above her pubic bone.

"What the fuck are you doing? Get off of me!"

"I'm so sorry," I told her, "but your baby is stuck and this is an emergency. I need to do some extra things to get your baby out and if you push it can be worse, so—"

"Don't let my baby die! Is he going to die?" her husband asked. At that moment I heard the sound indicating that the phone was beginning to record a video.

"I need everyone to be quiet and listen to me. Vanessa, look me in the eye. It's just you and me. This sucks, but I need you to stop pushing while I try to move your baby into a better position. OK?"

Eye contact made. It was just the two of us in the room.

"OK," she said.

"I'm trying a rotational maneuver," I called out to the nurse who had come in to help and track times. After a moment I added, "It's not working. I'm going for the posterior arm."

I reached my left hand in and felt for the baby's wrist. It slipped. Vanessa was crying, but her nurse was up in her face, coaching her to not push. The husband continued to record, and at that moment I couldn't stop to care about it.

I reached again, and this time I got the wrist. I was able to sweep the arm across the chest and deliver the arm. Baby's top shoulder was now free.

"Vanessa, push with everything you have."

She did, and a huge baby was born. He had the audacity to be totally fine and came out screaming, even as I was trying to slow my own pulse. The husband yelled into the phone, "Look at my baby! He is perfect!"

Our timekeeper nurse called out, "Time of dystocia, fifty-two seconds." Of course, she had to be wrong, since it was at least an hour and a half—because that was how it felt to me.

Vanessa hopped off the table and said, "OK, how did we all think that went?"

This was a simulation of a shoulder dystocia. And as much as I hated every minute of it because it felt so real (the model, the actors, the screaming), it's also why I love these simulations. We practice these emergencies so that when they happen in real life, we are prepared to provide the best care we can.

But some people *definitely* missed their calling in acting.

I'M PRETERM AND HAVING COMPLICATIONS, BUT I'M NOT READY TO HAVE A BABY YET!

I assure you your team doesn't want you to have your baby early unless it's absolutely needed, or unless they can't do anything to stop it. But there are a few reasons you might need to deliver before your due date:

1. You're in preterm labor that can't be slowed down or stopped.
2. Your baby isn't growing well (or at all).
3. Your baby is showing signs of distress in the uterus.
4. Remaining pregnant is too dangerous for *your* health (i.e., high blood pressure, bleeding, needing medical treatment where remaining pregnant would be too dangerous).

If this is happening to you, here are some questions you can ask that might help you feel more prepared:

1. Why are you recommending I give birth now? Is there an option to wait and reevaluate, or is that not safe for us?
2. Is there a NICU here that can care for my baby, or will they have to be transferred to a different hospital?
3. *(If the answer to #2 is yes)* Can I be transferred so I can deliver there? If not before birth, can I be transferred after? Or is that too dangerous for my own health currently?
4. Can I talk to the pediatric team to know what to expect from having a baby born this early?
5. Can I still try for a vaginal birth?
6. If my baby is in the NICU and I can't meet their needs with my own breastmilk, do you have access to donor milk?
7. What is the NICU visitation policy?
8. Do you have child life support to help me explain this to my other children?

It can sometimes feel like you are blindsided when you are told you are about to meet your baby weeks or months before you thought you would. It's OK to feel all the feelings and fall apart while you process it. Just know that there is a lot of support out there for parents in your same situation, and many people who will help you through this.

HELP, MY BABY IS BREECH! NOW WHAT?

I want you to take a deep breath and know that while this might feel unexpected, you've got this.

Lots of babies start out breech (with their butt or foot down) but eventually turn to the head-down, ready-for-birth position. Only about 4 to 5 percent of babies remain breech at full term. So if you've been told your baby is breech at your twenty-week anatomy ultrasound or a thirty-two-week growth ultrasound, I would encourage you to realize that this is normal—don't panic.

SOME TERMINOLOGY TO HELP WITH THIS SECTION . . .

ECV: External cephalic version

TOLAC: Trial of labor after cesarean

VBAC: Vaginal birth after cesarean

Head entrapment: When a breech baby's head is stuck in the uterus after the body has delivered through a cervix that isn't yet completely dilated.

Umbilical cord prolapse: An umbilical cord that comes out of the cervix before the baby is born. It can get compressed and cut off the flow of blood to the baby. The treatment is usually an emergency C-section.

Placental abruption: When the placenta detaches from the wall of the uterus before the baby is born, which can result in life-threatening bleeding and decreased blood flow to the baby.

If you're nearing your due date and your little one is still breech, though, it's time to consider your options. Those include:

	What it is	Pros	Cons	Dr. Jen's notes
Doing nothing, and delivering by C-section	Undergoing a scheduled C-section, usually around 39 weeks of pregnancy	• You have a plan and a date • You don't expose yourself to the risks of an external cephalic version (described on page 149) or vaginal breech birth	• Requires a C-section, and the risks that go with it (for more, see page 33, "Can I just request a C-section?") • You may go into labor before then and need your C-section sooner • Makes future pregnancies slightly higher risk • If you don't have a provider who offers a trial of labor after cesarean (TOLAC), then you may be signing up for future repeat C-sections.	• Totally acceptable if this feels right for you—just consider your goal family size (one and done, or five?) and what repeated C-sections may mean. • If you may want to aim for vaginal births in the future, see if your provider is on board.

	What it is	Pros	Cons	Dr. Jen's notes
Doing nothing, and opting for a breech vaginal birth	Delivering your breech baby vaginally	· No recovery from surgery · No future risks from having a C-section	· Not commonly offered in the United States due to increased risks to baby and lack of training. More on this below! · Complications like head entrapment and umbilical cord prolapse can occur and harm the baby.	I would only consider this at a center and with providers that do these regularly and with proper evaluation, preparation, and clear consent.
Trying at-home ways to get your baby to flip	This can include moxibustion (a Chinese medicine technique that involves burning an herb near your little toe with the idea that it stimulates your uterus and your baby turns in response), pelvic tilt maneuvers, or acupuncture.	· Probably very little harm in trying · Can give you a sense of control and doing something that may feel less invasive than an external cephalic version	· You can burn your toe with moxibustion if you aren't careful! · Acupuncture may be costly if not covered by insurance.	Data shows that moxibustion may help compared to doing nothing, so I think it's great to try if you're interested. There's no good data to show the other methods work, but it doesn't mean you can't give them a whirl!

	What it is	Pros	Cons	Dr. Jen's notes
Trying an external cephalic version (ECV)	This is where we try to turn your baby into the head-down position by guiding them with our hands. We use an ultrasound to assess if it is working and to check your baby's heart rate during the procedure.	• Works about 50–80% of the time • If it works, avoids a C-section for a breech baby	• Can be painful if you don't have anesthesia. • Risks include placental abruption (0.2%) and needing an emergency C-section (less than 1%) if your baby doesn't tolerate it. • More common is a temporary drop in your baby's heart rate (occurring about 10% of the time), but almost all of these resolve without needing an emergency C-section, as described above.	• I love a good trial of an ECV because it can help someone avoid major surgery, but if it freaks you out, it's OK to skip it. • If your provider doesn't mention using anesthesia, ask! A spinal can help with the pain, and it increased the success rate from 37% to 60% in one study!

Whatever you choose, it's important to feel like you have a choice in how you birth. If you're wondering why C-sections seem to be the norm and not a vaginal breech birth, the main reason is that a large study from 2000 showed results that concerned many of us in our field. Content warning: It's talking about neonatal death, so I do want to call out that it can be hard to read.

This study reported that bad outcomes like death and serious injury were much higher in breech babies born vaginally (5 percent) as compared to those born by C-section (1.6 percent). However, follow-up studies showed that the vast majority of breech babies born vaginally were fine years later—meaning if they did not die during birth or shortly after, they were at no greater risk than babies born via C-section.

All of this is to say most OB-GYNs (and even midwives) don't offer vaginal breech birth because of this study, fear of litigation, and lack of training. That said, it doesn't mean you can't find a provider who feels skilled in offering this, and if that's something you might be interested in, it's worth a conversation with your team.

MY BABY'S HEART RATE IS WORRYING MY LABOR TEAM—WHY IS THIS HAPPENING?

Decels.
Lack of variability.
Tachycardia.
Bradycardia.
Lates.
Deep variables.

These are all words you might hear us say, and it might sound like another language—but it is how we describe various patterns that we see on fetal heart-rate monitoring (see page 95, "Talk to me about fetal monitoring").

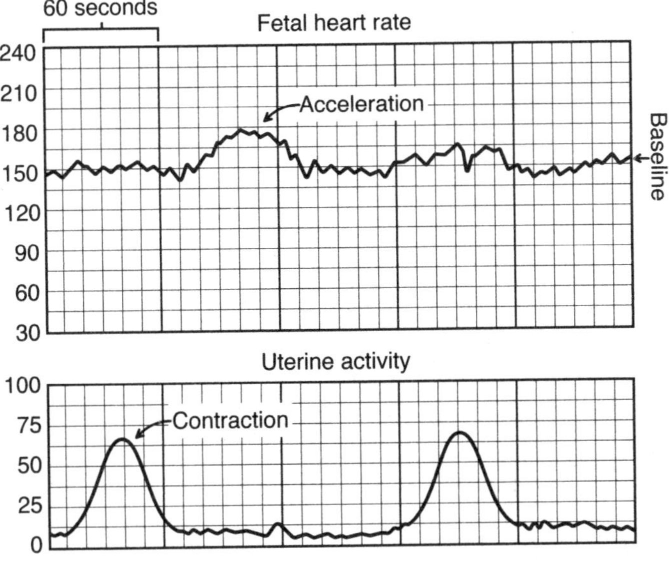

Fetal heart rate and uterine activity tracing

When your nurse, midwife, or doctor says that your baby's heart rate is worrying them, what they might mean is:

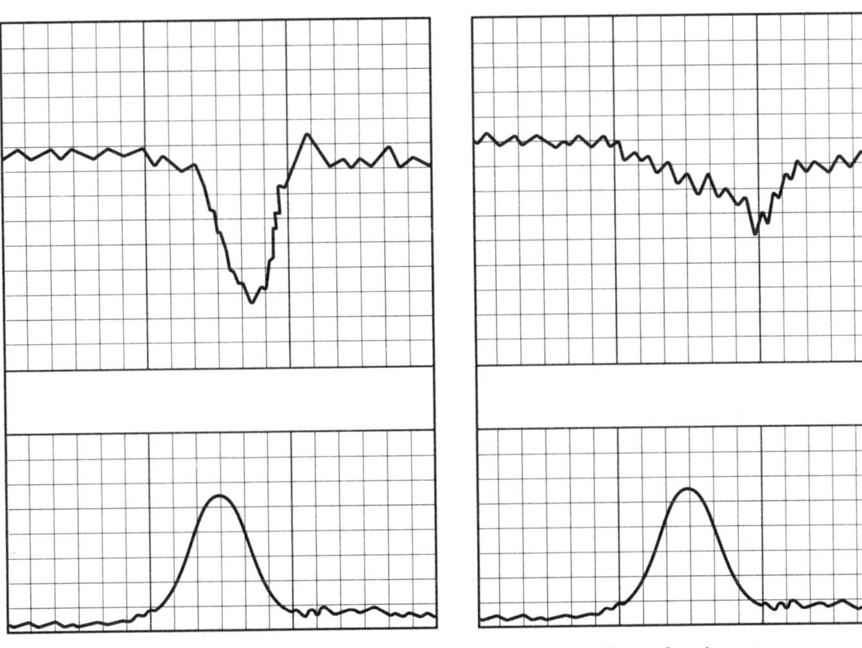

Variable deceleration

Late deceleration

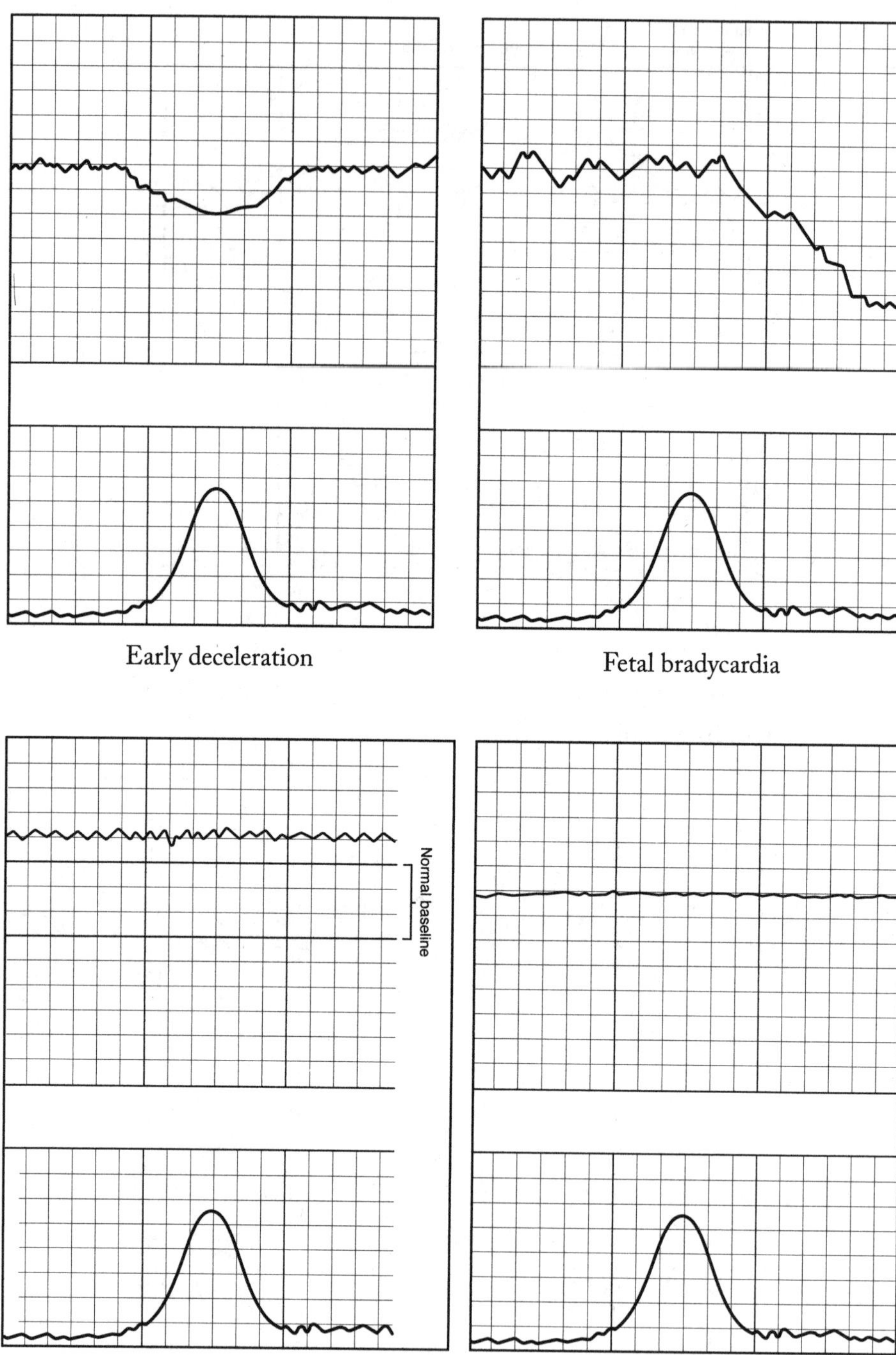

Early deceleration

Fetal bradycardia

Fetal tachycardia

Minimal variability

What we say	What we see	What it means	What we might suggest or do
There are decelerations (decels) present.	Dips below your baby's baseline heart rate. There are different kinds of decelerations; some are worrisome, and some are not at all.	It depends on the type, but it can mean: • The cord is getting compressed (variables). • The placenta isn't transferring oxygen well (lates). • The baby's head is getting squished as they move down the birth canal (early decels).	• Nothing (if it's not worrisome). • Position changes (to help get baby to move and stop putting pressure on their cord). • Putting fluid via a catheter into the uterus to give more cushion to the umbilical cord (called an **amnioinfusion;** see page 98, "And they want to put monitors . . . inside of me?"). • Stopping Pitocin or giving medicine to decrease contractions. • Recommending a C-section if it's very concerning.
It's too flat.	Your baby's heart rate is flatter than we'd like and lacks variability (small variations up and down in the tracing of the heart rate that look like small squiggles).	• It can be normal if it's time-limited (and is just your baby taking a short nap) or if it is the result of certain medications we use in labor. • If it's more prolonged or it's completely flat, this can be a sign your baby isn't getting enough oxygen.	• Nothing. • See if your baby wakes up with stimuli—whether using our fingers to touch their head during a cervical exam or using a device called an **acoustic stimulator** (literally like a vibrator we put on your belly; we expect the noise and vibration to wake them up). If they respond with more variability in their heart rate, we know they're just fine. • Stopping Pitocin or giving medicine to decrease contractions. • Recommending a C-section if it's very concerning.

What we say	What we see	What it means	What we might suggest or do
It's too low.	The baseline of your baby's heart rate is lower than normal (normal for a baby is usually above 110 beats per minute). This is called bradycardia.	It could be that we're monitoring your heart rate and not your baby's. It could also be a side effect of medications, a sign of distress like placental abruption (placenta separating from the uterus too soon), an issue with your baby's heart (this is rare), a deceleration that is beginning, or . . . it could be completely normal.	• Check your pulse to make sure we aren't picking up your heart rate. • Continue to monitor if we aren't worried it's something to be concerned about. • Measures described above if we think it's a deceleration, including an emergency C-section if it's a sudden and dramatic heart rate drop.
It's too high.	The baseline of your baby's heart rate is higher than normal (i.e., above 160 beats per minute). This is called tachycardia.	This can be the first sign of an infection in the uterus (called chorioamnionitis—more on page 171, "Why do I have a fever in labor?") or fever in the mom or baby. It can also be a side effect of certain medications or drugs, very rare uncontrolled thyroid problems, and more rarely issues with the electrical wiring of the baby's heart.	• Check for signs of infection (checking your temperature, seeing if your uterus is tender). If an infection is confirmed, Tylenol and antibiotics are often started, and this can fix the baby's high heart rate. • Giving IV fluids. • Reviewing medications and your medical history to see if there is a treatable cause. • Continuing to monitor if other signs are reassuring. • A C-section may be recommended if the fever is very high, lasts a long time, or there are other concerning signs.

As you can see, it's not always straightforward. If your team has concerns, you can get more information by asking:

1. What is it you are seeing that worries you?
2. What do we think the cause is?
3. How worried are you?
4. How can we make it better?
5. What would be a sign we need to deliver my baby right now?

I WAS TOLD I HAVE HIGH BLOOD PRESSURE AND I'M SCARED.

You are far from alone in having a diagnosis of high blood pressure (hypertension) in pregnancy or in feeling worried by it. With up to 8 percent of pregnant people experiencing this (and that number is only increasing), this is something your OB-GYN or midwife is very experienced in diagnosing and managing.

High blood pressure in pregnancy comes in a few different flavors, so the first thing to know is which one you have:

Diagnosis	When it happens	Blood pressure	Lab tests	Symptoms
Chronic hypertension	Diagnosed before or in the first 20 weeks of pregnancy	· ≥ 140 (top number), ≥ 90 (bottom number), or both · Two measurements four hours apart (usually)	Normal	None
Gestational hypertension, without severe features	Diagnosed after 20 weeks of pregnancy		Normal	None
Gestational hypertension, with severe features		≥160 (top number), ≥110 (bottom number), or both	Normal	None
Preeclampsia, without severe features		· ≥ 140 (top number), ≥ 90 (bottom number), or both · Two measurements four hours apart (usually)	May have an abnormal level of protein in your urine and/or other lab test abnormalities like low platelets, decreased kidney function, or abnormal liver function	None (you may notice sudden weight gain or swelling in your hands and face, which you should tell us about, though it's no longer formally part of how we diagnose preeclampsia)
Preeclampsia, with severe features		≥160 (top number), ≥110 (bottom number), or both	Lab tests that are even more severe/abnormal than above	May include: · Headache · Pain by your liver · Vision changes · Trouble breathing · Abnormal heartburn, nausea, or chest pain
HELLP (**h**emolysis, **e**levated **l**iver enzymes, **l**ow **p**latelets) **syndrome**		· ≥ 140 (top number), ≥ 90 (bottom number), or both · Two measurements four hours apart (usually)	· Diagnosed when labs are at their most abnormal levels · Most severe form of preeclampsia	

You may have received one of these diagnoses earlier in pregnancy, or the first time it might show itself is when you are in labor (or even postpartum). The overall goal with all these is to avoid harm to you while balancing a potentially early birth for your baby.

One of the main things we are trying to avoid is the development of **eclampsia,** which is the most severe form of any of these disorders and is characterized by seizures. It can happen in about 1–4 in 200 people who have preeclampsia. Eclampsia can lead to brain injury, stroke, long-term disabilities, and even death. This can happen in pregnancy, during labor, or even in the postpartum period, which is why your team will be monitoring you closely and why they may recommend some of the interventions above.

Here are some recommendations we may have once you've been diagnosed with high blood pressure in pregnancy:

Diagnosis	What we may recommend	What the team is worried about	Dr. Jen's notes
Chronic hypertension	· Delivery often between 38 and 39 weeks (sometimes earlier if it's severe) · Closer blood pressure monitoring · Lab tests to evaluate for preeclampsia · Medications if blood pressure spikes · Continuous fetal monitoring · Staying a few extra days postpartum so you can be monitored more closely	· Risk of progressing to preeclampsia · Increased risk of damage to your heart, brain, or kidneys (rare overall, however), leading to issues like stroke and heart attacks · Increased risk of poor fetal growth and stillbirth · Increased risk of placental abruption	Chronic hypertension can become preeclampsia in 20–50% of pregnant patients, hence the increased monitoring during your pregnancy and recommendation for induction. We call this **superimposed preeclampsia.**

Diagnosis	What we may recommend	What the team is worried about	Dr. Jen's notes
Gestational hypertension, without severe features	• Delivery by 37 weeks or at time of diagnosis (if diagnosed later) • All of the measures above	Same as above, with increasing concern if severe	Up to 50% of people who have gestational hypertension will eventually develop preeclampsia, with the associated risks—hence the recommendation to be delivered sooner.
Gestational hypertension, with severe features	• Delivery by 34 weeks or at time of diagnosis (if diagnosed later) • All of the measures above		
Preeclampsia, without severe features	• Delivery by 37 weeks or at time of diagnosis (if diagnosed later) • All of the measures above • Steroid injections (medication to help your baby if they're less than 34 weeks) may be recommended, but sometimes we don't have time to wait to give them if you are very sick	• Same as above, with increasing concern if severe • Risk of developing preeclampsia with severe features, HELLP syndrome, or eclampsia	A medicine called magnesium sulfate may be used to decrease the risk of eclampsia, but data is unclear if it helps in this group. This is described more in the box on page 160.

Diagnosis	What we may recommend	What the team is worried about	Dr. Jen's notes
Preeclampsia, with severe features	• Delivery by 34 weeks, sooner (if very sick), or at time of diagnosis (if after 34 weeks) • All of the measures above • Magnesium sulfate infusions to decrease your risk of eclampsia • May require the input/ management of a high-risk OB-GYN specialist	• Same as above • High risk of complications makes staying pregnant beyond 34 weeks very concerning	It may seem too early to deliver, but these diagnoses can be serious if not managed properly.
HELLP syndrome	• Delivery at time of diagnosis, which may be very preterm • All of the measures above • May require blood product transfusions • May require intensive care unit (ICU)–level care	Same as above	
Eclampsia	• Delivery at time of diagnosis, once medically stabilized • All of the measures above • Additional antiseizure medication may be needed	Permanent brain injury and death	

WHAT IS UP WITH THAT MAGNESIUM DRIP?

Magnesium sulfate is an IV medication we use to decrease the chance you'll go on to develop eclampsia. It's just like the magnesium you already have in your body. We know it cuts your risk of eclampsia in half if you have preeclampsia with severe features, but if you have the non-severe variety the data isn't as clear. It *definitely* has some nasty side effects (hot flashes, nausea, drowsiness), and if the levels of magnesium go too high, it can cause heart and lung issues. This is why when you're on it we'll be watching you closely and at times monitoring your blood levels if needed.

One last thing before we move on: Many people have heard that the "cure" for preeclampsia is delivery. While we often focus on how we need to induce your labor to "fix" the problem, there is so much more to this story. While it's true that having your baby is the first step in resolving preeclampsia (because the culprit—while not totally understood—is actually a combination of how the placenta attached to your uterus, the blood flow from the placenta to your baby and you, and genetic and immunologic components), we know it can still cause issues postpartum and actually increases your risk of cardiac issues for the rest of your life.

This is meant not to scare you but instead to empower you: **Every person who has had high blood pressure or preeclampsia in pregnancy or postpartum should make sure their primary care doctor knows so your heart health can be monitored more closely over the course of your lifetime.** In the Resources section (page 297) I've included a link to a critical document you should print for you and your primary care doctor so they can know how to monitor your health moving forward after a preeclampsia diagnosis.

One final note: Preeclampsia can show up for the first time or flare again after your baby is born. Watch out for these signs of postpartum preeclampsia:

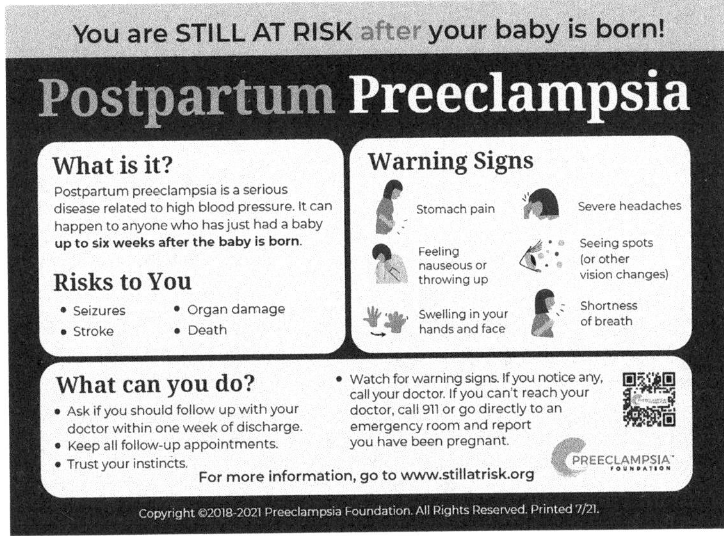

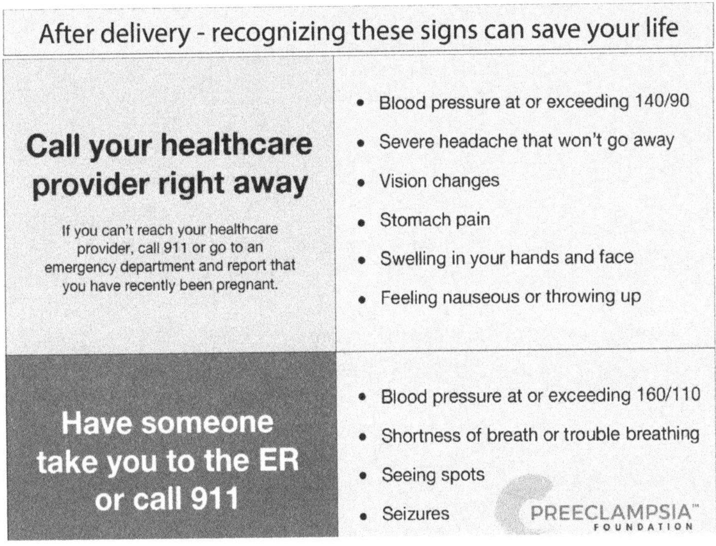

I'VE STARTED BLEEDING TOO MUCH—WHAT'S GOING ON?

This can be scary, but I want to assure you that this is something any OB-GYN or midwife is well-versed in managing—we see this often! Here's what can be some of the causes:

IN LABOR			
	What it is	**Common signs**	**How we treat it**
Placental abruption	The placenta separates prematurely from the wall of the uterus, causing bleeding. This happens in about 0.5% to 1% of pregnancies (higher if certain high-risk conditions exist, like preeclampsia).	• New bright red bleeding (may be a lot or a little) • Blood-tinged amniotic fluid when your bag of water breaks • May have contractions that are very close together (blood irritates the uterus) • Sudden drop in your baby's heart rate • If a lot of bleeding, your heart rate may increase and your blood pressure may drop	• If this is suspected and there is not too much bleeding and your baby's heart rate looks fine, we can continue the labor process and watch closely • If it's more severe and endangering you or your baby, we may need to do an emergency C-section • You may need a blood transfusion
Uterine rupture	The wall of your uterus opens up, either along a previous C-section scar or without prior history of surgery.	• Sudden intense abdominal pain • Sudden drop in your baby's heart rate • Baby moves higher up in the birth canal or into your belly • Often heavier vaginal bleeding	• Emergency C-section • May require hysterectomy (removal of uterus) if the rupture is large or involving large blood vessels
Torn vaginal or cervical tissue	Tissue may tear during vaginal exams or as labor progresses (example, if a piece of hymen remains and stretches and tears in labor).	• Often not very much blood seen • We can often see where the bleeding is coming from	• Applying pressure • Stitches • Often no therapy is needed

POSTPARTUM			
	What it is	**Common signs**	**How we treat it**
Torn vaginal or cervical tissue	Also called a **laceration,** this often happens during vaginal birth (cervical lacerations are less common). These are described in more detail on page 200, "How do I prevent tearing?"	• Can be seen after giving birth	• If bleeding or deep, lacerations will be repaired with stitches that dissolve after a few weeks • If a larger tear or your provider needs to be able to see better, this may be done in the OR • More info on page 217, "What happens if I need stitches?"
Uterus isn't contracting down	Called **uterine atony,** this is when the uterus doesn't contract back down after you give birth, which is the main way the uterus clamps off bleeding blood vessels.	• Ongoing vaginal bleeding after birth • Uterus feels "boggy" and not firm • Uterine size increases (meaning it is filling with blood)	See next page for more

POSTPARTUM			
	What it is	**Common signs**	**How we treat it**
Retained placenta	A piece of the placenta remains in the uterus, which prevents it from contracting down.	· As above · Part of the placenta may be missing when examined · Can be seen on ultrasound as well	· **Manual removal:** Your doctor or midwife will reach in and remove the placental piece (yes, we can use pain medication!) · **Curettage:** We use a tool to scoop out the remaining placenta (if you've heard of a "D&C" it's the "C" part) · **Hysterectomy:** If the placenta is abnormally attached to the uterus (such as a placenta accreta), the entire uterus may need to be removed · For more info, see page 213, "When (and how) does the placenta come out?"
Uterine inversion	The uterus turns inside out (I know; sorry).	· Can be seen in the vagina	· Your provider will use their hand to guide the uterus back in; rarely, surgery is needed to fix it
Bleeding disorders or conditions	Can be an inherited problem with blood clotting (like von Willebrand's disease) or as a result of other disorders, like HELLP syndrome.	· Often bleeding not only from the uterus but also anywhere a blood vessel is injured, like an IV site	· Blood test monitoring · Blood transfusions · Medicines to help with blood clotting · Possible transfer to ICU

I do want to expand on the treatment of **uterine atony**, since **this is the cause of up to 80 percent of all postpartum bleeding problems.** If your team suspects this, this is what they will almost always do:

1. **Massage the heck out of your uterus.** This is called fundal massage, but the truth is, it's no Swedish massage moment. It's literally one

of us using our hand to press down on your belly and rub your uterus with the goal of helping it contract down. We can also place our other hand in the vagina to help massage the bottom part of the uterus, called the *lower uterine segment,* which sometimes needs a little help firming up. We know it's annoying, but it can be hugely effective. Usually if you have an epidural, you often don't even feel us doing it, but if you do or if you have no pain relief on board, ask us! We can definitely give you something to help. We know it's working when your uterus starts to feel hard like a rock and your bleeding stops.

2. **Empty your bladder.** If your bladder is full, it pushes up against the uterus and prevents it from contracting down. We can place a small tube into the opening of your bladder to help get the pee out. We can either remove this immediately or leave it in (called a Foley catheter) if you're losing so much blood we want to keep a closer eye on you.

If you're *still* bleeding, we can do all or some of these interventions:

1. **Give medicine to help your uterus contract.** These are called **uterotonic medications,** and they do what they sound like: They help your uterus squeeze down. In most every hospital Pitocin is given, either in your IV or as a shot in your thigh, as your baby is born or just after to prevent bleeding. If you continue to bleed, this dose can be increased. If this isn't working, your team may use one of these extra medications:

Medication	How we give it	Dr. Jen's notes
Misoprostol (Cytotec)	Rectally, under the tongue, or swallowed	This is the GOAT of bleeding medications, as it works really well, can be given to almost anyone, and is cheap. Unfortunately, some states are making it harder for us to use this because of abortion bans (which is one way bans harm people who are trying to have kids, but I'll just stop there).
15-methyl PGF2α (Hemabate)	Injection into your thigh or (less commonly) the uterus itself	Can't be given if you have asthma.
Methylergonovine (Methergine)	Injection into your thigh	Can't be given if you have high blood pressure.
Tranexamic acid (TXA)	Given in your IV	Newest medicine on the block for postpartum hemorrhage.

Note: A common side effect of these medications is diarrhea, so you may be given medicine to prevent that. But don't worry if you poop. Pooping is better than bleeding.

2. **Sweep out any blood clots.** If your uterus is filling with blood, we can use our hand to sweep it out. The goal is to help the uterus get smaller and contract to stop further bleeding. We may use an ultrasound to see what's happening inside as well.

   If bleeding continues, now we up our response:

3. **Using a tool to physically help us.** If the above interventions aren't cutting it, we can place a device in the uterus as our next step. Two options currently exist:

   - **Vacuum device.** Also called the Jada System, this is placed in the uterus and then hooked up to suction to force the uterus to contract. It is often only left in place for an hour or two and then removed. I love this thing—it works really well.
   - **Using a balloon device.** This device (most commonly called a Bakri balloon) is placed in the uterus and then filled with water

like a balloon to press against the bleeding blood vessels of the uterus. It's usually left in place for up to twenty-four hours and then removed.

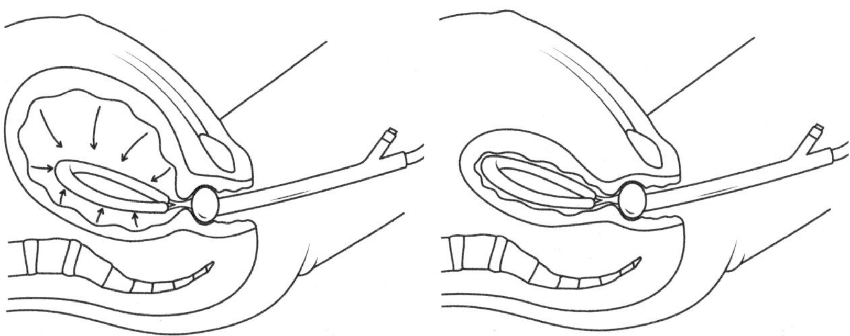

Jada vacuum device placement (left) and hooked up to vacuum suction (right)

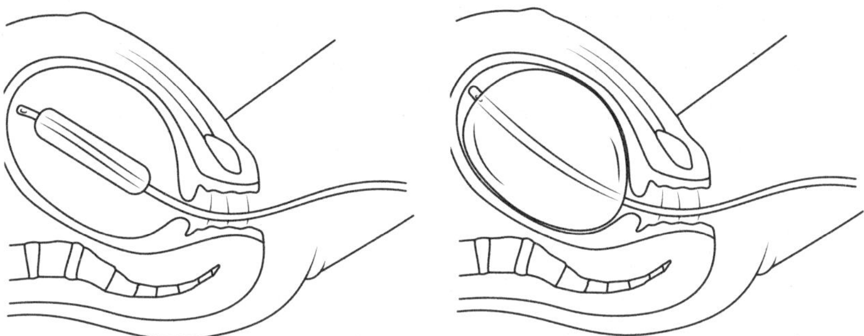

Bakri balloon insertion (left) and fully inflated balloon (right)

4. **Call our interventional radiology friends.** If bleeding continues but you are stable enough that you can be transferred to radiology—and your hospital has access to this—you can undergo a procedure called **uterine artery embolization.** This is where a radiologist will use X-ray imaging to see where your bleeding is coming from. They will then block off the blood vessels using coils or small beads fed through an incision in a blood vessel in your thigh. This can avoid the loss of your uterus, but it can make your future pregnancies higher risk as well as make getting pregnant potentially more difficult. This is usually not available at smaller hospitals.

5. **Proceed to surgery.** This may be tried sooner if you've delivered by C-section and are still in the OR, if we're really worried about your clinical status, or if your hospital lacks some of the above options. Depending on your bleeding, your OB-GYN can use stitches to stop the bleeding or help compress the uterus. If those fail, we can remove the uterus entirely (**hysterectomy**). We don't usually jump to this first, as removing a recently pregnant uterus is not easy and can have more complications associated with it than your standard hysterectomy.

This section included a *ton* of information—and that was intentional. Since this complication is pretty common, and I've often seen how in the moment it can be scary and confusing, I wanted to give you a road map to understanding what your team might or did do.

If some of this happened to you, I am sorry. It can be traumatizing, so head to page 272, "I think I had a traumatic birth and I don't know where to go for help," if you want tips on how to process this.

WHAT IS A SHOULDER DYSTOCIA?

This is when your baby's head delivers but one of their shoulders gets stuck (often under your pubic bone). This requires a few extra maneuvers to help dislodge that shoulder and help your baby arrive safely.

Shoulder dystocia can happen in up to 3 percent of all births, and while some risk factors exist (like having a bigger baby or having diabetes in pregnancy), the vast majority of shoulder dystocias occur in people with no risk factors. This is why we are always prepared to manage this emergency and practice it often via standardized medical simulation!

The good news is that *most* shoulder dystocias are brief and are fixed with a few quick maneuvers, leaving no permanent complications for mom or baby. The bad news is that sometimes they last longer (think five to ten minutes), require multiple attempts at delivery, and can result in long-lasting issues.

What's so bad about being stuck? Here are some of the complications we are trying to prevent:

1. **Brain injury.** Being squished like this can decrease the amount of oxygen getting to your baby. The longer this goes on, the worse it usually is. The good news is that this happens in less than 1 percent of all babies who experience a shoulder dystocia.

2. **Nerve injury.** This often happens in baby's arm (called a brachial plexus injury) when the nerves get stretched. It can happen spontaneously even in routine births or be the result of pulling too hard while that one shoulder is stuck. Most of these injuries are temporary, though some can be permanent.

3. **Bone fracture.** Sometimes we do this on purpose to help your baby be born (yes, really—see below), but occasionally the collarbone or one of the arm bones may break during delivery. I know it sounds scary, but these heal amazingly well, often without any issues.

4. **Worse tearing or bleeding for you.** Whether from the size of your baby or us needing to do extra maneuvers to help get your baby out, lacerations that are more severe can definitely occur, and they may lead to more blood loss. For more on this, see page 217, "What happens if I need stitches?"

So how do we manage a shoulder dystocia? Here are some things we can do. It's important to note that there's no one-size-fits-all or one order to try these in—this is where the experience and expertise of your doctor or midwife come into play:

1. **Recognize you've got a shoulder dystocia.** This sounds obvious, but your provider will see the shoulder is stuck, let everyone know, and call for help to get extra folks in the room. Warning: It will feel like

a million people are in your room because it's all hands on deck when we have emergencies!

2. *Stop pushing.* This might sound counterintuitive, but you continuing to push as your doctor continues to pull on a baby with a stuck shoulder is what can lead to worse nerve injuries.

3. **Get you in a better position.** This might include dropping the head of your bed down flat, flexing your legs back (called the **McRoberts maneuver**), or having you get on hands and knees (called the **Gaskin maneuver**) to make more room for your baby.

4. **Push above your pubic bone.** Your nurse might push here to try to guide the stuck shoulder out. This is called **suprapubic pressure** and sometimes is all that is needed to get your baby across the finish line.

5. **Reach in and grasp the bottom arm.** Your provider can reach in with one hand to help guide out the bottom arm—doing this makes more space for that top one to come under the pubic bone. This works really well and is personally my favorite maneuver, but it's not always possible if you don't have an epidural or we can't get our hand in there because of the size of the baby or shape of your pelvis.

6. **Rotate that baby!** There are several techniques where we can guide your baby to rotate and help that stuck shoulder loosen up. They have names like the **Rubin maneuver** or the **Woodscrew maneuver** and involve us placing our hands on your baby's shoulders to try to get them in a better angle to be born.

7. **Perform an episiotomy.** The goal here is to make more space to allow our hands to perform the maneuvers above. These aren't done routinely or needed in many shoulder dystocias, and you can read more about them on page 203, "Will I need an episiotomy?"

8. **Purposely fracture the clavicle.** Trust me, no one wants to break a bone in your baby, let alone do it on purpose. But sometimes we

need to if the above measures haven't worked and we need to make that diameter of your baby's chest smaller to get them out safely. The good news is these fractures often heal up amazingly well without any issues if done correctly. Also, this is pretty rare.

9. **Proceed to surgery.** Let me just say that this is hardly ever done (so feel free to stop reading), and if we are here, this has been the worst shoulder dystocia your OB-GYN has ever seen. This is where we push your baby's head back in and then proceed with a C-section. As you can imagine, the amount of time this takes often means a baby may not do well or survive this.

If you're reading this because you've had a shoulder dystocia in a prior birth, talk with your doctor or midwife about plans for your future deliveries. Sometimes a C-section may be recommended to try to avoid this happening again, but this is an individual decision, and one best made with a team that can review what happened and take your concerns into account.

WHY DO I HAVE A FEVER IN LABOR?

Quick refresher: A fever is defined as a temperature of 100.4 degrees F (38.0 degrees C) or higher. Fevers in labor can be due to any of the following:

1. **Side effect of medication.** Some medications, like misoprostol, can have fevers as a side effect. It's not a true "fever" per se, but likely a result of the drug interacting with the thermoregulatory centers in your body.
2. **Side effect of an epidural.** This can be seen in up to 25 percent of people who get an epidural, with the cause being what was mentioned above as well as the epidural causing a (noninfectious) inflammation.

3. **Infection in your uterus.** This is the one we worry about—more below!

4. **An infection elsewhere.** Things that can cause a fever in anyone (a cold, GI bug, COVID, or other illness) can still be in play when you're in labor.

If you've had a single temperature reading that indicates a fever, your team will take additional steps, which could include some or all of these:

1. Taking your temperature again to see if it's truly elevated.
2. Doing tests to look for signs of infection in your body, such as bloodwork, nasal swabs, or a urine sample.
3. Doing an exam to see if your uterus is abnormally tender, which could indicate an infection.
4. Monitoring your baby's heart rate more closely.

A uterine infection in labor is called **chorioamnionitis** or **intra-amniotic infection.** This means there could be an infection in the amniotic fluid, placenta, uterus, or baby. We treat this with IV antibiotics since this infection puts you and your baby at some increased risks, which can include:

- Abnormal labor progress (an infected uterus doesn't work as well)
- Postpartum hemorrhage
- Sepsis (a severe infection in your bloodstream that can affect your organs); this can happen in both you and your baby

The good news is that your obstetric team is very used to diagnosing and treating fevers in labor. If antibiotics were given, we will usually continue these after you give birth if you deliver by C-section, or if you were very sick and birthed vaginally.

The pediatric team will watch your baby for signs of infection once they arrive—this can range from the usual newborn care to doing tests for infection to admitting them to the NICU and giving antibiotics. What is done will depend on the clinical circumstances and how worried they are about your baby, so don't hesitate to ask for an explanation if some of these treatments are recommended.

I do want to highlight that **a fever or even a diagnosis of a uterine infection is not on its own a reason you must deliver by C-section.** Your team may recommend one if they have other concerns as well, such as your labor isn't progressing or you're getting very sick despite antibiotics, but I want to reassure you that many people with fevers in labor go on to have successful vaginal births.

WHAT HAPPENS DIFFERENTLY FOR TWINS? TRIPLETS?

So. Many. People!

If you've had multiples, then you know what I'm saying is true: When we're expecting more than one baby to arrive, it feels like a spectator sport given the number of people who are in the room at the time of delivery.

How your babies come out is a discussion between you and your obstetric team. For triplets (or more) we almost always recommend delivery by C-section, though I have known of a few people who've had triplet vaginal births. When it comes to twins, delivering vaginally or by C-section will depend on their position, size, gestational age, the experience of your provider, and your desires.

Here's what else you can expect if you're carrying more than one baby and it's their big day:

Extra monitoring	Two babies means two heart rates to watch, so your belly will be covered in monitors. And tracing these babies can sometimes be tricky, so your nurse might spend quite a bit of time chasing them and adjusting the monitors, or you may have one monitor placed internally to assist in this (see page 98, "And they want to put monitors . . . inside of me?").
An extra IV	Being pregnant with multiples increases your risk of some complications, like heavy bleeding. Because of this, your provider will likely recommend you have not one but two IVs in case an emergency arises.
Discussion of an epidural	If you're planning a vaginal birth, your team may discuss their recommendation for an epidural (rather than being neutral on this, as we usually are). This is because if you need something called a breech extraction or an urgent C-section, an epidural can make these more comfortable and safer.
Having your babies in an operating room	Even if you're having a vaginal birth, many hospitals will recommend that anyone with multiples delivers in an OR in case an urgent C-section is needed. (We can make this less sterile-feeling by dimming the lights, playing music, and more, so don't hesitate to ask for this if it's important to you!) You may start pushing in your labor room and then move to the OR when you're getting close to birth, or head to the OR first, before you start pushing. It can depend on your team, if you've had babies before, and whether your babies are preterm.
A big crew	Like I mentioned above, more people are present. Each baby has their own pediatric team, so that's double (or triple) the people. An extra OB-GYN is also usually present to help with ultrasound guidance and for safety, as well as an anesthesiologist in case a C-section is needed.

MY [INSERT NAME OF PERSON YOU CAN'T STAND HERE] IS HERE AND I WANT TO KICK THEM OUT. CAN MY NURSE HELP ME DO THIS?

Oh yes, they can!

Listen, we are here to help you have the birth you want and deserve. We have *zero* problems running interference between you and visitors who are getting in the way of that. We can also do this in a way that doesn't put you in the middle, such as stating that visiting hours are over, or that you need to rest, and everyone needs to leave.

If this feels awkward or you know there's going to be that person who shows up despite you wishing they hadn't, here are some tips I've seen work really well to advocate for yourself:

1. Ask your OB-GYN or midwife to put in a prenatal visit note something like this: "Patient's mother not to be allowed in labor room. Please notify admitting desk that if she shows up, patient is not accepting visitors."
2. Ask for a note to be posted on your door that states "No visitors" or "Check in with nurse before entering."
3. Most times your nurse will ask all visitors to leave the room to complete your admission paperwork. This is a great time to go over concerns like this.
4. Ask your nurse to help you to the bathroom. Once in there and it's just the two of you, let them know who you need to have leave, and they can make it happen.
5. Come up with a safety phrase. You can let your nurse know that if you say, "I'd like some apple juice," that means you want her to ask all visitors to leave, or just the one person who you've got concerns about. This might seem ridiculous, but guess what? It works really well.

6. If you're worried about people calling and getting information about whether or not you are in the hospital, let your team know this. They can change your name in the computer system so that it is protected, and you'll be there anonymously.

7. In more extreme cases, if people aren't leaving despite our requests, know that we can gladly go up the chain of nursing supervisors and security. You are our priority, and we won't tolerate visitors who get in the way of that.

I HAD A TRAUMATIC BIRTH BEFORE AND I WANT TO KNOW HOW TO HAVE A BETTER EXPERIENCE THIS TIME.

I am so sorry your prior birth resulted in trauma. Sometimes people ask me what constitutes a traumatic birth, and my response is always the same: If you felt traumatized, mentally or physically, then that counts. I cover this more on page 272, "I think I had a traumatic birth and I don't know where to go for help."

I think it's important to call that out because what may be traumatic for one person may be perfectly fine for another, and vice versa. This isn't the Trauma Olympics, and whatever happened, let's focus on having this not happen again.

Here are some tips I recommend to prepare for your next birth experience:

1. **Let go of the guilt.** Lots of feelings can bubble up after a traumatic birth: guilt that you somehow caused it, or regret that you didn't see something coming or speak up when you were concerned. It is OK if you didn't know what you didn't know, because now you're experienced—and this can be empowering. Now we can take that

experience and use it to plan for the birth you need, want, and deserve this time around.

2. **Identify what happened last time.** This sounds simple, but I want you to get super granular. Was it needing a C-section? Or was it not the C-section itself but the feeling of being rushed and not heard? Was it a specific person? Was it a lack of understanding of what was happening? Or was a specific wish blatantly ignored?

3. **Think about what you need this time around.** This may involve working through this with someone qualified, like a therapist. Do you need to make sure you are heard better, or your pain is not ignored, or certain words are not used? Do you want everything explained to you, or do you just want others to take the wheel? There are no wrong answers here.

4. **Do you need a new provider?** Was an issue with your OB-GYN or midwife insurmountable and you deserve to see someone who treats you better? Or do you love your OB-GYN, but you need her to advocate on your behalf to get the postpartum support you didn't get the first time around?

5. **Tell your team what happened.** If you feel comfortable doing so, discuss what happened last time with your OB-GYN or midwife during your prenatal care, to make sure they get it and they know what you need to go right this time around. Share it with your labor nurses, too. When we know how we or the system failed you last time, we can do our very best to make sure it doesn't happen again.

6. **Have advocates in your corner.** Whether it's a doula, your partner, or friends or family members, employ them to speak up and be your voice if you aren't comfortable or aren't able to.

7. **Make a birth plan/preference.** See page 44, "Should I make a birth plan . . . or does every OB-GYN hate them?" When you've had a traumatic birth, a written plan that highlights what happened and what you need this time around can be very empowering. As an

example: "I was forced to deliver on my back last time, and I felt a lack of control. I want to birth in whatever position feels best and is safe for me and my baby."

It's important to note that any birth may require pivoting if there are concerns or unexpected surprises, including a birth where we are trying to not have a repeat of prior trauma. Even if a change in plan happens despite your having detailed conversations with your team, it's important to know your team should be able to pivot in a way that is still respectful and informed.

I PLANNED A HOMEBIRTH AND HAVE TO TRANSFER IN; WHAT SHOULD I KNOW?

Common reasons for a hospital transfer:

- Wanting pain management
- Concerns over your baby's heart rate
- Increased bleeding
- Labor that has stalled
- Lack of progress with pushing
- New-onset high blood pressure
- Retained placenta
- Need for a complicated vaginal or cervical tear repair

You're probably having a lot of feelings: Fear of the unknown. Disappointment. Concern that you'll be judged. I get that, as I'd be lying if I didn't acknowledge that we haven't always made transferring to the hospital feel easy or judgment-free.

As someone who has accepted many transfers from home and birth centers, I want you to know that **you deserve to be treated with respect.** I also want you to know that I have been lucky to be part of some wonderful births that started at home but ended in the hospital, and everyone involved left healthy and satisfied with the way the story played out.

Here's what I want you to know:

1. Go back to page 20, "I'm going the homebirth/birth center route—what now?," to revisit questions and answers that hopefully you've reviewed during your pregnancy.
2. Confirm that your homebirth midwife has contacted the hospital you'll be transferring to. This ensures they have rooms available and will know of your arrival and can be prepared.
3. Ensure that your midwife has faxed your prenatal and labor records or plans on hand-delivering them to the hospital team.
4. Ask your midwife to accompany you to the hospital. While they likely won't be able to be involved in the medical care once you are admitted to the hospital, being there in person means they can answer all questions regarding what's happened up until this point. They can also stay on in the doula or support role if that's allowed.
5. Ask to be transferred to the care of a hospital midwife. This can often feel less daunting, and I've seen this play out well many times. Some situations may not be appropriate for this, such as when a C-section is clearly needed or you have a higher-risk pregnancy or labor, but if that's not the case, it never hurts to ask.
6. Communicate what's important to you. Having a hospital birth plan can be helpful in these scenarios, but if you don't have one, that's perfectly OK. Pick someone from your support team to speak up on your behalf about the things that matter most to you. It might be "She wants delayed cord clamping and to deliver standing up. How can you support us in that?"

7. If you are feeling judged for your choice to deliver at home, feel free to be blunt and let people know that this isn't acceptable. If you notice one particular nurse, midwife, or doctor who is making you feel this way, ask to speak to someone about finding a replacement (sometimes this isn't feasible, but it's OK to ask).

8. You can still have a vaginal birth in many cases, but sometimes it means using interventions that you hadn't planned on, like Pitocin or an epidural. Know that it's OK to feel sad if your plan veered off course, and feel free to acknowledge this with your team while also accepting certain interventions if it feels right.

9. Coming into the hospital doesn't mean staying there—I've had homebirth patients who've come in to have a vaginal tear repaired only to go home an hour or so later and finish their postpartum recovery at home with their midwife.

THE GRAND ENTRANCE (OR EXIT)

SO MANY BIRTHDAY PARTIES

One of the best parts of my job is seeing the birth of not just a baby, but a family—and how different that can look from room to room.

I have been a part of babies arriving in so many different ways:

- In a room crowded with cheering family members, including a few on FaceTime
- With everyone in a hush because the two-year-old big sister finally fell asleep on the couch, only to wake up once that baby comes out crying to say, "Oh, my brother is here!"
- Into the peaceful atmosphere of dim lights, battery-powered candles, and a jazz soundtrack
- With Ozzy Osbourne blasting from the operating room speakers
- To be shown to their dad to announce the baby's sex, only for me to say, "No, that's a vulva!" when he panicked in the moment and got confused
- To parents who have navigated loss who now see their healthy baby, and finally exhale
- In the hallway, because some babies don't wait
- Via gestational carrier (surrogate) where everyone in the room has tears in their eyes
- To a teenager who I know is going to make a wonderful parent, despite what others may think
- In less than sixty seconds from the start of a C-section under general anesthesia where everyone in the room holds their breath until we hear that baby's cry

Each birthday party is unique, and I am so lucky I get to be invited to so many. But I know it can be scary not having any idea what yours might be like, so I hope this section sheds some light on what you can ask for, what you can expect, and more.

MY NURSE SAYS IT'S TIME TO PUSH. HELP!

Congrats, you're almost there! But holy crap—you are about to push something the size of a watermelon out of your vagina. Your fear is valid . . . and I think this stems from the unknown, the horror stories we see online, and the fact that things are about to get very real.

So. Let's combat the unknown part and talk about pushing.

As I discuss on page 116, "What is the best position to labor in?," **you don't have to labor or give birth on your back unless there's a medical reason your team has shared with you.**

You also don't *have* to push as soon as your nurse, midwife, or OB-GYN says your cervix is completely dilated and it's time to go. However, I do want to highlight that the concept of delayed pushing or **"laboring down"**—which is where someone doesn't push right away and instead lets the fetus come down passively in the birth canal, with the idea that this saves energy, shortens pushing, and increases the chances of a vaginal delivery—is actually no longer recommended. Newer data shows us that doing this increases rates of postpartum hemorrhage, infection, and low oxygen in babies.

It's always your choice, though, and there's definitely a difference between taking a few moments to get your mind wrapped around pushing versus waiting two hours to begin.

With that in mind, I need you to know that successful pushing is:

1. What feels acceptable to you
2. Is tolerated by your baby
3. Appears to be working

Notice how I didn't say that one position was best? It's because it's not, and I cover it more in the next section. Your team can give you feedback, and I'd really encourage you to keep an open mind if your nurse (who will be by your side the entire time you're pushing, often while your doctor or midwife will come and go) thinks a position or technique might need a change to work better. And by "working" I mean your baby is moving down in the pelvis and their heart rate shows us they aren't minding the squeeze.

Here's how I've seen parents birth their babies:

1. Taking a deep breath in, holding it, pushing for ten seconds, and repeating this three to four times with each contraction (this is called the **Valsalva maneuver**).
2. Pushing like the above, but doing it with every other contraction.
3. Laughing/sneezing/vomiting their babies out (usually not the first baby . . .).
4. Screaming/moaning/breathing their babies out and never once "bearing down" in a coached way ("open glottis").
5. Pushing on your back, your side, on hands and knees, with a sheet in tug-of-war style, on a toilet, standing up, and any number of other ways (more on this in the next section).

I want to really emphasize keeping an open mind when it comes to this part of labor. You may have envisioned birthing on hands and knees without coached pushing only to not have much progress after two hours. If your midwife suggests a trial of Valsalva pushing on your side, consider giving it a go and seeing if it helps. Sometimes the method you least expect to work is the one that does it!

WHAT IS THE BEST POSITION TO PUSH AND DELIVER MY BABY IN?

If you say on your back, or standing, or squatting: You're wrong!

I say that because there's no one best position. The real answer is that the best position to birth your baby in is the one that you want to be in, that is safe for you and your baby, and that seems to be working. I said it before, but it's worth repeating because I see so many misconceptions about this in the labor room and online: The real "best" position can mean different positions for different people.

Whenever I make a social media post showing a birth simulation where my model is shown on its back, I always get comments like "You should never birth on your back! It's the worst!" I get what people are trying to say—that no one should be *forced* to birth on their back. That there may be times when this actually makes it *harder* to get the baby out. And that many OB-GYNs like myself were trained with this as the default, so we tend to think of this as the best position. I completely agree with these statements.

The reality is that **studies show birthing positions like standing, squatting, side-lying, being on all fours, or sitting on a birthing stool or toilet can be better than lying on your back or semi-upright.**

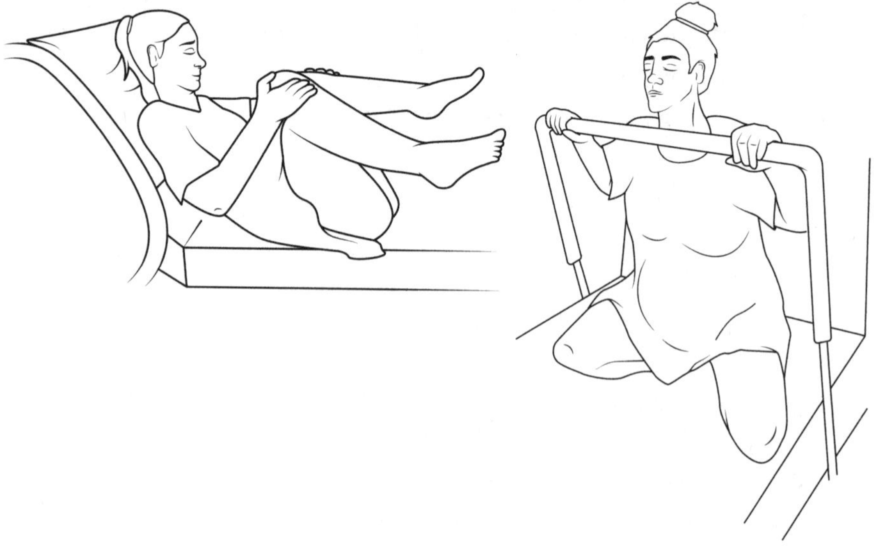

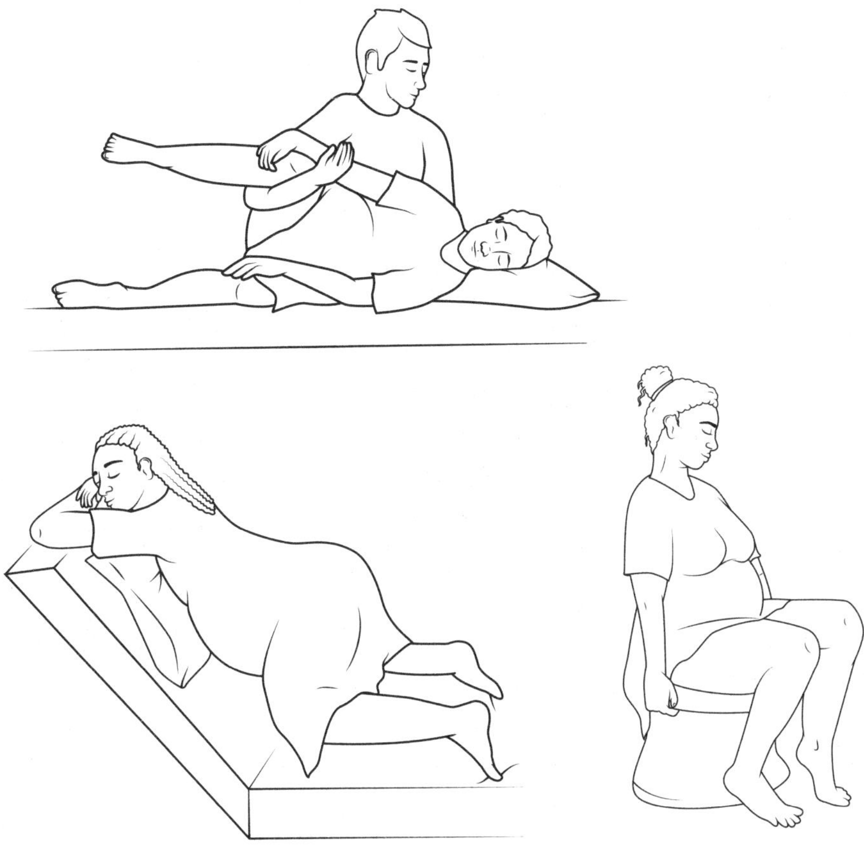

When I say better, I mean that for those **without an epidural** you can expect:

- Slightly shorter time spent pushing (about five to fifteen minutes less)
- Lower rates of needing a forceps or vacuum delivery
- Less pain
- More vaginal tears, but lower episiotomy rates

The caveat is that you might lose more blood when birthing upright (though studies disagree). But if you do, you won't lose so much that it outweighs the potential benefits of being in these positions.

For those **with an epidural,** the evidence isn't as clear, but **birthing on your side and changing positions regularly in labor** are likely helpful. I think the side-lying part makes intuitive sense, as this takes pressure off your tailbone and allows it to open up more, giving your baby more room to come down and out of the pelvis.

So what should you do if you want to birth in a position that isn't on your back and you're worried your birth team won't have it? First, discuss this *before* you're in labor. If your provider tells you they don't "allow" any other position than being on your back, well . . . I think you know what I'm going to say. This is your body and your birthday party, and you get to have a voice in how that party goes down.

It can also be helpful to pass along that the following organizations have all agreed that you should be supported in the birthing position that *you* choose:

- American College of Obstetricians and Gynecologists
- World Health Organization
- American College of Nurse-Midwives
- Midwives Alliance of North America
- National Association of Certified Professional Midwives
- Association of Women's Health, Obstetric and Neonatal Nurses

Second, understand that there may be times your team may *need* you on your back if it's truly a safety issue. If you have severe preeclampsia and have dangerously high blood pressure that gets worse if you stand up, they may not want you upright. If you need a forceps or vacuum delivery, almost all doctors (myself included) will need you on your back, as this is a technical procedure that we need to do in the way we are trained best.

If you think you might want to birth in a non-lying-down position, I highly recommend taking a birth class to see your options in action and know what's available to you. If you can, hire a doula (see page 31, "Do I need a doula?") who can be with you to support your plan and be a voice and an advocate.

And remember this fun fact: Babies can be born in almost as many positions as they can be made. *wink wink*

HOW LONG IS PUSHING GOING TO TAKE?

How long you push depends on a few factors, such as:

- If you've delivered vaginally before
- The size of your baby
- Their position in your pelvis at the start of pushing
- Whether or not you have an epidural

That said, the average time people will push and give birth vaginally according to the most recent data we have is:

First baby	
Without an epidural	About 45 minutes
With an epidural	About 1.5 hours
Second baby or more	
Without an epidural	About 15 minutes
With an epidural	About 30 minutes

These are just averages, and I want you to know that **it can absolutely be normal to go beyond these times** (ranging from two to even four hours in some cases). These averages are also not a time limit after which we tell you that you must have a C-section.

For more on what is considered prolonged pushing and how we might manage that, head to page 127, "They say my labor is going too slowly—what does that mean?"

WHAT IF I POOP? PEE ON MY DOCTOR? THROW UP?

This is just another day at the office for us—I can't stress enough how much we really aren't fazed by these natural parts of labor.

If you're worried about having your support people around to witness this, though, I would use this as a good measure for deciding who you want in the room when you give birth. If it feels too awkward to have them see you poop, then you might want to reconsider having them present for this part.

And about pooping: We actually get excited when this happens. No, not because we are weird, but because it shows us that you're pushing in the right way that will get your baby out. So, we really do mean it when we say, "Push like you're pooping!" or "You're pooping, that's great!" (OK, maybe we are a little weird.)

Your team can also help you not feel embarrassed in these moments by using washcloths to wipe anything that comes out, or helping you rinse your mouth if you throw up. We won't let anyone take pictures during these moments!

THEY'RE TELLING ME I NEED A C-SECTION BUT I DON'T THINK I NEED ONE. CAN I SAY NO?

You can say no to anything (remember, I cover that on page 137, "What am I allowed to say no to?"), but it's important to be informed so you can understand what saying no might mean for you or your baby. If you feel this way, I recommend asking questions first so that you can make an informed decision.

The first thing you should do is ask why they're recommending it. C-sections might be suggested for one of the following reasons:

1. Your labor has slowed down or stalled.
2. Your baby's heart rate looks concerning.
3. You've been pushing without any progress.
4. You are sick and need to have your baby sooner rather than later.
5. Your baby is not head-down.
6. Your baby is large. *(This is controversial! More on this below.)*
7. You're pregnant with multiples.
8. You're bleeding a concerning amount.
9. The umbilical cord has prolapsed into your vagina.
10. You have a history that makes it more likely that the uterus will rupture in labor (for example, you've had more than two C-sections, or you've had some types of uterine surgeries).
11. The placenta is covering or very close to the opening of your cervix.
12. You have an active genital herpes infection.

I cover why a C-section may be recommended for a slow labor on page 127, "They say my labor is going too slowly—what does that mean?," as well as options for breech babies on page 146, "Help, my baby is breech! Now what?"

But I do want to address the idea that a C-section might be recommended if your baby is on the bigger side. This is generally done to avoid the risk of a shoulder dystocia (discussed on page 168, "What is a shoulder dystocia?") and severe vaginal tearing and hemorrhage. You might hear the terms "large for gestational age" or "macrosomia." These mean:

	How it's diagnosed	Definition
Macrosomia	In pregnancy by ultrasound	The fetus weighs more than 4,000–4,500 grams (8.8–9.9 lbs)
Large for gestational age	After birth when baby is weighed	A birth weight at or over the 90th percentile for gestational age

Fun fact: In the United States, 7.8 percent of all newborns weigh more than 4,000 grams, and only 1 percent of all newborns weigh more than 4,500 grams.

But not all large babies are created equal, meaning some absolutely can be born vaginally without a C-section being needed. So how do we decide who we recommend a C-section to for having a "big baby"?

General expert guidance suggests that we discuss having a scheduled C-section for babies who on ultrasound:

- Weigh more than 4,500 grams (9.9 lbs) if you have gestational or preexisting diabetes.
- Weigh more than 5,000 grams (11 lbs) if you don't.

We use the lower weight cutoff for pregnant patients with diabetes, since we know these babies carry their weight a bit differently and the risks of shoulder dystocia for them are higher.

I want to clarify that these aren't hard-and-fast rules. To be honest, our ultrasounds are not 100 percent accurate, but especially if growth has been consistently large over multiple ultrasounds, it's an important discussion to have with your provider.

In the end, any recommendation for a C-section should be made for evidence-based reasons that weigh the risks and benefits of pursuing this versus continuing to labor. If your team doesn't seem worried and they let you know you can have more time to decide, use this time to chat with your support team and get your questions answered. You can use the Q&A guide on page 15 to help guide you.

WHAT IS A VACUUM OR FORCEPS, AND WHY MIGHT I NEED IT?

Sometimes babies come right out, and sometimes they don't and need some assistance. Forceps and vacuums are devices that can help guide a baby out of the birth canal when they or the person pushing need a little help. These are used in just over 3 percent of births in the United States.

Forceps are metal tongs that are placed around the baby's head, while a vacuum uses direct suction. This might sound gnarly, but when used for the right reason and in trained hands these can be lifesaving tools with very little risk and excellent results—a healthy baby, born vaginally!

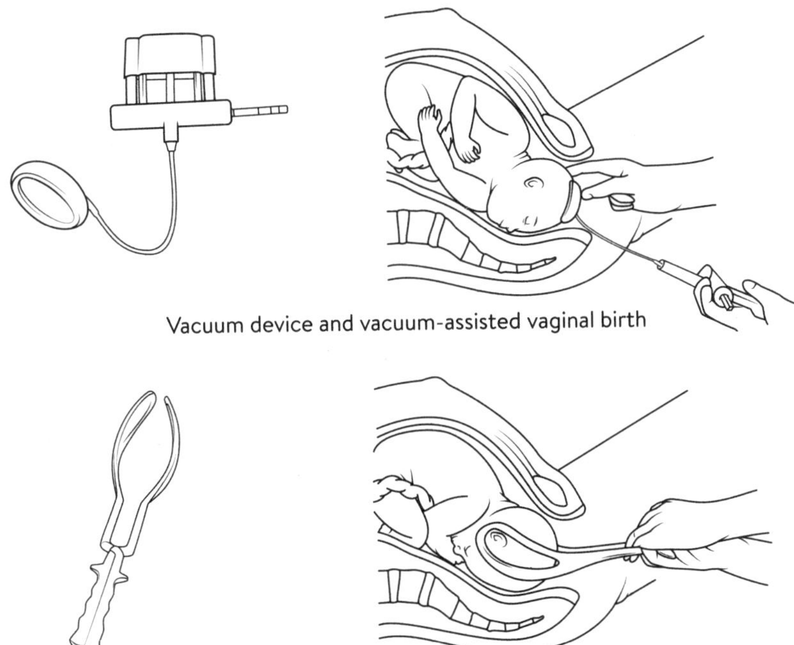

Vacuum device and vacuum-assisted vaginal birth

Forceps and forceps-assisted vaginal birth

These types of births are called **operative** or **assisted deliveries,** and reasons they might be used are:

1. You've been pushing for hours and are exhausted.
2. Your baby's heart rate is of concern and your team is worried they need to be born quickly.
3. You have a medical condition where pushing is too dangerous (such as certain cardiac conditions).
4. You've been pushing for a while, but your baby is not moving down any lower.
5. Your baby's head is a little cockeyed and needs to be rotated to fit better.

The benefit of having an assisted delivery is that you have a good chance of avoiding a C-section, which may be the alternative. If your provider suggests this, you may want to ask how urgent it is, what the alternatives may be, and what method they'd recommend and why.

Most doctors have a preference for one device over the other because that's what they've been trained to use, and in this scenario it's almost always better to go with the one they are the most comfortable (and therefore successful) using. This can be great to know and clarify long before they might be used—such as during your prenatal care or on admission, if it's a new doctor you haven't seen before.

However, I would be doing you a disservice if I didn't review the pros and cons of these tools so that you can make an informed decision. I don't want the table below to freak you out, so I ask that you keep the following in mind: Risks do exist, but it's about balancing them against the alternative. C-sections have their own risks, and sometimes a C-section can't be done quickly enough to prevent a concerning outcome in your baby. If we have this concern, we will strongly recommend that they need to be delivered ASAP, likely via a vacuum or forceps if that is possible.

	Forceps	Vacuum
Success rates	Higher	Lower (but depends on the user)
Vaginal and/or rectal tearing	Higher risk	Lower risk (but higher than an unassisted delivery)
Bleeding in/around baby's brain	Same risk (about 1 in 650–850)	
Urinary/stool leakage or overactive bladder symptoms in the future	Some studies show same risks for both, while others show a higher risk using forceps (up to 20% risk of overactive bladder compared to 10% for a spontaneous vaginal birth, and 10% risk of leaking urine at one year compared to 3% for vacuum/spontaneous birth).	
Pelvic organ prolapse in the future	Vaginal birth itself is a risk factor (30% by fifteen years), but it is increased by using forceps or vacuum (45%). Forceps are more often to blame because the pelvic floor muscles are more likely to be injured with them, leading to prolapse.	
Postpartum pain with sex	One study showed a higher risk compared to unassisted vaginal birth (14% compared to 4%)	No increased risk in that same study
Need an episiotomy to do successfully?	No! Should not be done routinely. More on page 203, "Will I need an episiotomy?"	
Risk of lacerations on the face, facial nerve injury, eye trauma	Higher risk because of where the forceps are placed, but still low risk overall (for example, about 0.9% for nerve injury, almost all of which recover on their own)	
Risk of scalp laceration, bleeding under the scalp, or around the brain or eyes		Higher risk because of where the vacuum is placed, with severe bleeding rare at 0.6%

In the old days, forceps were used almost routinely and mainly to benefit the OB-GYN, not the patient or baby. Today we are more aware that while they can work wonderfully, there are some risks associated with their use, and so they should only be used when needed, and only with full informed consent and agreement. The same can be said for vacuum-assisted deliveries, or any obstetric intervention.

MY BABY IS "SUNNY SIDE UP" AND I AM NOT SURE WHAT THAT MEANS.

This refers to how your baby is situated in your uterus and pelvis. The medical term for a sunny-side-up baby is "occiput posterior" (OP). That is, their occiput, or the back part of their skull, is facing your posterior, or back. (The typical presentation is occiput anterior, or OA—the back part of their skull is facing your front.)

A picture is worth a thousand words, so let me show you what we mean:

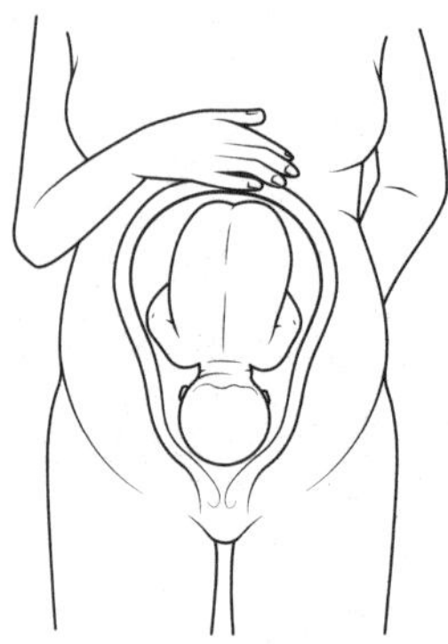

Occiput anterior (OA)

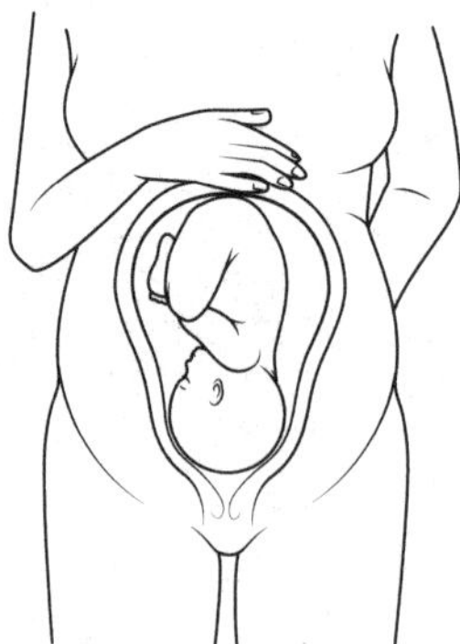

Occiput transverse (OT)

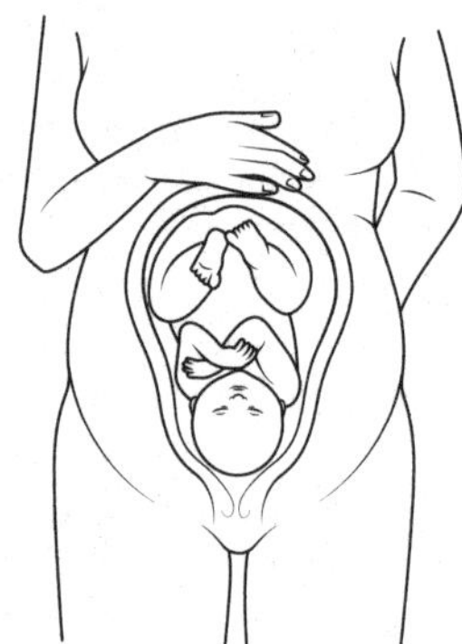

Occiput posterior (OP)

Why might your provider mention this? Because we know that having a baby that stays in the OP position can increase your risks of:

1. Needing to deliver by C-section
2. Needing an assisted delivery with forceps or vacuum
3. Having a more painful labor
4. Worse vaginal tearing
5. Increased risk of postpartum hemorrhage

All of this is because this position makes it a bit harder for your baby to navigate the pelvis since a larger diameter of the head has to fit through. I find this picture really helpful in understanding why:

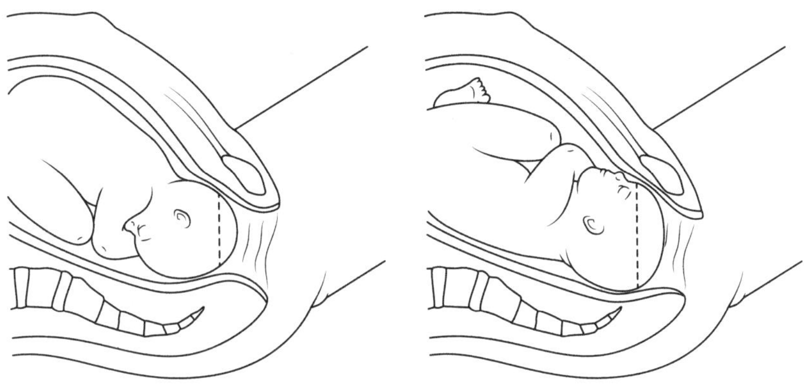

The smaller head diameter in the baby in the OA (left) position can be seen as opposed to the baby in the OP (right) position.

That said, before you start to worry about which way your baby is looking, let me share the top six facts you need to know about having a baby in the sunny-side-up position:

1. **This is *normal* before and in the early stages of labor.** So don't be freaked out if on an ultrasound on your admission for induction

your baby is OP! Up to one-third of all babies are OP in the early stages of labor.

2. **And of those, most will rotate to OA as labor progresses.** About 95 percent of babies move into the OA position on their own, and this makes sense, as it's easier for them to fit into the birth canal this way.

3. **You *can* have an OP baby vaginally.** It is not a reason for a C-section by itself, and I've had many patients birth babies in this position just fine. However . . .

4. **If it's causing trouble, we can try to help your baby turn.** Sometimes being in the OP position can slow labor down, but there are some things we can do to try to get your baby to rotate. Certain position changes in labor can help encourage your baby to rotate. I highly encourage you to use the resources at Spinning Babies (page 298) for more on this. Doulas are often trained in these techniques too, so that's yet another reason to consider having one! We can also try something called a **manual rotation,** where we insert a few fingers or our hand in your vagina to try to turn your baby.

5. **But the key is not to intervene too soon.** If your provider is going to try to manually rotate your baby, it's important to wait until you're fully dilated to give your baby the chance to do it on their own. Whether to do it before you've begun pushing versus after you've pushed a while (and progress is absent or slow) is still up for debate. But we *do* know that current data suggests manual rotation can decrease your need for a C-section without increasing risk to you or your baby. It's more comfortable with an epidural, so you might want to consider that if your doctor or midwife is recommending it.

6. **Persistent OP babies can cause more painful labors.** We often hear our patients talk about more back pain (back labor) when there's a sunny-side-up baby involved. This is likely because your baby's

spine and body are pushing against your own spine more intensely in this position. Doing those positional moves described previously can help with relief and get your baby into a less uncomfortable position, but also know that it's OK to ask for pain medication if you need it.

WHAT WILL IT FEEL LIKE WHEN THE BABY COMES OUT?

Here's what I've heard people describe what it felt like to them:

- "I felt nothing—my epidural was great!"
- "I felt like I was being ripped in half."
- "I felt like I was pooping a really big poop."
- "Everything was burning. It was like my vagina was on fire."
- "It was the worst pain of my life, and then it was gone once she was out."
- "I only felt pain on one part of my belly where my epidural wasn't working."

There are as many descriptions for what someone feels during birth as there are stars in the sky—and they're all true! For my first birth, for which I had an epidural, I felt pressure but no pain. With my second, no epidural, I remember the contractions being intensely painful . . . but the actual delivery part felt like this huge moment of relief.

I will say that this obviously depends on whether you use pain medicine such as an epidural, other options I have listed on page 107, "Ow! I'm in pain! What can I do?," or nothing, as well as your own pain tolerance.

In general, most people without an epidural will say that this shit hurts. And it does, generally in four different ways:

1. **Contraction pain.** Contractions can be intensely painful . . . but then you get a break once one subsides.

2. **Crowning.** This is when the baby's head delivers. Many people describe it as a "ring of fire" as those nerves stretch. This is when I usually hear the most four-letter words.

3. **Delivering your baby's shoulders.** This is when we will often ask you to push strongly, and it can either hurt or not depending on how easily your baby comes out.

4. **Delivering your placenta.** This usually feels like intense pressure or pooping that is then followed by a sensation of physical relief. Placentas don't have a head or shoulder, for which I am intensely grateful.

HOW DO I PREVENT TEARING?

Up to 80 percent of people who birth vaginally will have some kind of laceration or tear. I know this might make an "abdominal bypass" sound like the way to go, but the good news is that the vast majority of these tears are small and easy to fix with stitches, or even no repair at all. ("Abdominal bypass" is maybe one of my favorite nicknames for a C-section, second only to "using the sunroof"—and I have former patients to thank for both of these hilarious euphemisms for what really is a major surgery. More on that on page 129, "Talk to me about C-sections.")

Back to being serious: Wanting to know how to minimize your risk of tearing in your vagina, on the perineum (the skin between the vulva and anus), and the rectum is totally valid.

Not all lacerations are created equal, so we use a grading system:

1. **First degree:** involves only the skin
2. **Second degree:** involves the skin and underlying muscle
3. **Third degree:** involves the skin, muscle, and all or part of the anal sphincters
4. **Fourth degree:** involves the skin, muscle, sphincters, and anal skin (i.e., through the rectum)

Here are interventions I often get asked about, including what the evidence says (or doesn't):

Intervention	This means . . .	Evidence shows . . .	Dr. Jen gives this . . .
Perineal massage in pregnancy	Starting at 34 weeks, using a lubricated finger (yours or a partner's) to gently stretch the bottom half of your vagina (imagine a clock: from three o'clock to nine o'clock) for a few minutes a few days a week	• It may reduce tearing if it's your first birth, likely because it decreases the rate of episiotomies. • Not as much benefit if you've delivered vaginally before.	A thumbs-up if it's your first time birthing vaginally, but only if you want to do it (some find it uncomfortable) and if you don't *overdo* it—that can cause more trauma to the area!
Perineal massage in labor	Performing massage while pushing or in between pushes	Has been shown to decrease third- and fourth-degree lacerations.	A thumbs-up (only with your consent, of course).
Perineal support in labor	Using a "hands-on" technique to support the perineum as well as also using a hand on the baby's head to control the delivery	The jury is out, as studies are conflicting, but a hands-off "no touch" method is acceptable and may be better.	It's a toss-up, and really the experience of your provider likely comes into play here. But stay tuned if we get better data!
Warm compresses while pushing	Using a warm washcloth on the perineum while pushing	Has been shown to decrease third- and fourth-degree lacerations.	A thumbs-up.

Intervention	This means . . .	Evidence shows . . .	Dr. Jen gives this . . .
Birthing in positions other than on your back	Birthing while standing, squatting, on hands and knees, or lying on your side	• Without an epidural: May increase risk of second-degree tears but decrease risk of third- and fourth-degree tears. • With an epidural: Side-lying was shown to have far less risk of tearing.	• Without an epidural: Consider staying off your back to prevent more severe tears, but also do what feels right overall. • With an epidural: Big thumbs-up for side-lying!
Having a midwife and not an OB-GYN	What it sounds like!	Midwives are less likely to use episiotomies as well as forceps or vacuum, which may be why their rates of lacerations can be lower.	Your choice, with the most important factor being who you choose and how they manage birth. Ask about episiotomy and severe tear rates no matter who you pick.
Having an episiotomy	Making an incision with scissors to create more space, with the idea to prevent worse natural tears	No evidence to support doing this routinely, with known harm if done unnecessarily.	An enormous thumbs-down—more in the next section.

Here's the quick summary of the most evidence-based choices from the table above:

IN PREGNANCY:

- Perineal massage if it's your first

YOU DON'T HAVE AN EPIDURAL:

- Try to stay off your back
- Warm compresses while pushing
- Perineal massage while pushing or in between (if you can tolerate it)
- No routine episiotomy

YOU HAVE AN EPIDURAL:

- Side-lying
- Warm compresses while pushing
- Perineal massage while pushing or in between
- No routine episiotomy

If I can give one piece of advice, it's this: No matter what you choose from the techniques above, when your baby is crowning, try to breathe your baby out and aim for a gentle, calm, controlled delivery. Birthing this way, rather than a dramatic popping out, can be more controlled and potentially lead to less tearing.

"THEY WANT ME TO USE A MIRROR?"

Yes, it's true that we have mirrors on stands that you can use when pushing to guide your efforts and act as some major motivation! It's OK if the idea of seeing down there is not for you, but I've had some patients who've loved it. It's also been super helpful at the end to help you "breathe" your baby slowly out.

WILL I NEED AN EPISIOTOMY?

Most likely not.

An episiotomy is when we make a small cut at the vaginal opening to make it wider. This is done to make more room for the baby to come out and can help a vaginal birth happen more quickly. It can also be recommended to potentially prevent worse natural tearing, but this often isn't needed.

There are two kinds, which you can see below. **Midline episiotomies** can be associated with higher rates of extending into lacerations that can go through to your rectum (more on this in the previous section), while **mediolateral episiotomies** are associated with more bleeding and increased pain with healing.

It's an intervention, so it's important to know the benefits as well as the potential risks:

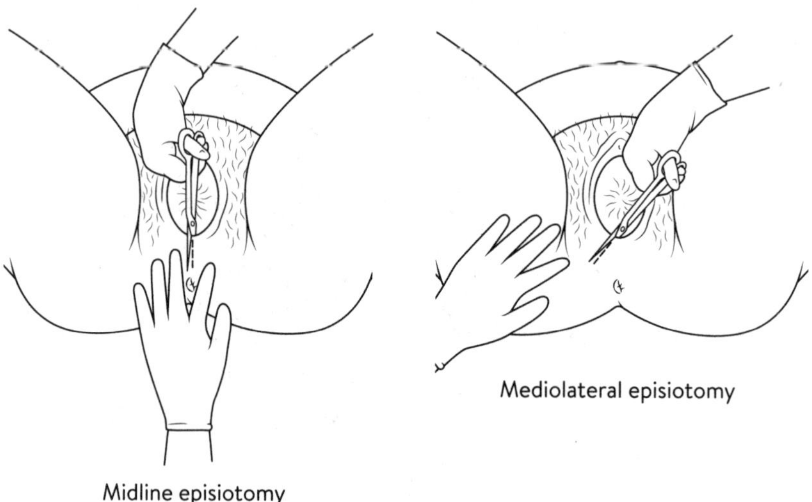

Mediolateral episiotomy

Midline episiotomy

Risks	Benefits
Increased pain with healing	Shortens time to delivery
Potentially increased blood loss (depending on the type of episiotomy)	Can be useful in a shoulder dystocia
Potential increased risk of urine and stool leakage (incontinence)	Can be useful for some vacuum and forceps deliveries
Slower return to sexual intercourse	

Episiotomies used to be done almost routinely for most births—in the 1970s they were performed in more than 60 percent of all vaginal deliveries!—because doctors believed it prevented worse tearing, was easier to repair than natural tearing, and protected the pelvic floor muscle during forceps deliveries. Let's be honest: It also was done because some doctors were impatient.

I am happy to report that we no longer think like this, and the World Health Organization, the American College of Obstetricians and Gynecologists, and other leading groups all agree episiotomies should *not* be routinely done and instead used only when necessary, given their potential risks.

That "when necessary" should really be reserved for cases such as:

1. Your baby is very close to being born but is showing signs of distress, and an episiotomy can make delivery happen more quickly.

2. There is a shoulder dystocia and your provider needs more room to do maneuvers to relieve it (more on page 168, "What is a shoulder dystocia?").

3. Your doctor is performing a vacuum or forceps delivery and needs additional space to place and maneuver the instruments (this is often not needed, FYI).

Data from U.S. hospitals in 2023 shows a national episiotomy rate of 4.6 percent, which is *much* better than those 1970s stats! I do want to flag that these rates vary and can still be unacceptably high in some hospitals or with some doctors. Data from 2015 showed rates as high as 40 to 60 percent still in some hospitals!

Here's what I recommend to be more informed when it comes to episiotomies:

1. Check your hospital's rate by choosing the "Maternity Tab" on this website and searching the episiotomy rates (**https://ratings.leapfroggroup.org**).

2. Ask your doctor or midwife about their *own* rate, as well as that of their practice if they may not be the one there at your birth.

3. Ask what kind of episiotomy they typically do if needed.

4. If it is being recommended in the moment, ask why and if it is truly necessary. Sometimes it's a true emergency, and if that's the case they should communicate that with you.

WHAT HAPPENS WHEN THE BABY COMES OUT?

Yay, they're here!

But do you ever wonder exactly what goes down in those moments? Shows have gotten better at depicting this more realistically (though I still laugh when a mom is handed an obvious two-month-old who's oh-so-clean and definitely not a newborn), but this is in general what you can expect:

1. Baby is born, hooray!

2. They are placed on your belly, either skin-to-skin or on a baby blanket.

3. The cord is left intact for at least one minute (more on why in the next section).

4. If your baby is vigorous and crying, awesome—this crying is great because it's opening their lungs and clearing fluid out.

5. If they aren't crying at all or very much, we will often try to encourage them to cry by rubbing their back or flicking their feet. This stimulation is often all they need to perk up, but if we have concerns, we may need to bring them over to the baby warmer to have

our nurses and pediatric team check on them and support them as needed (with some oxygen, deeper fluid suctioning, etc.).

6. If there's a lot of fluid in their mouths that we can see or hear (like they're gurgling), we'll use a bulb suction that gets the gunk out. We used to do this routinely; it's now only recommended as needed (and if done unnecessarily, it can cause a baby's heart rate to drop).

7. After a minute or more, two clamps will be placed on the cord close to your baby's belly button, and the cord will be cut in between these clamps. Your partner, other support member, or even you are welcome to do it—or we can. Just let us know.

8. Since your baby comes out rather wet, we will at this point switch out any wet blankets and cover them with a warm blanket while they remain chest-to-chest with you for ideally the first hour. We know this time is super important to help their transition to the outside world, and barring any medical issues for you or baby, this is the best place for them (if it's not possible, having your partner do this skin-to-skin contact is also a fantastic option). This is called the "golden hour," and I cover it more on page 219, "What is this 'golden hour' I keep hearing about?"

9. Your nurse may put a hat on your baby since the belief that babies lose lots of heat from their heads is still prevalent, despite lack of any real data to support this practice for healthy, full-term infants. In fact, hats can actually prevent you from smelling your baby, which has been shown to trigger more oxytocin release (the feel-good hormone that helps with breastfeeding and decreases your hemorrhage risk!), so feel free to pass on it if it's offered.

10. While your obstetric provider is busy delivering your placenta (which usually happens in the first few minutes after giving birth), the above will be happening and your team will also be checking out your baby right on your chest. They'll listen to the baby's heart and lungs and make sure they've got a good heart rate and temperature.

11. You'll have Pitocin started (or increased to a higher dose) once your baby is born or your placenta is out. We do this because it decreases your chances of postpartum hemorrhage. It can also be given as a shot in your thigh if you don't have an IV or it stopped working. You can choose to skip this, but I would say this is something that makes me a bit nervous, as it works well (see page 161, "I've started bleeding too much—what's going on?") and postpartum hemorrhage is not uncommon.

12. If you've had any vaginal tearing, your doctor or midwife will let you know if it needs to be stitched up; see page 217, "What happens if I need stitches?" You can keep your baby on your chest during this repair—in fact, I am a huge fan of this, as I call it "baby anesthesia"!

13. For the first hour or so after a vaginal birth, you'll be monitored more closely for bleeding and pain control. This means some extra blood pressure checks and something called **fundal massage**—which is not a massage at all but rather your nurse pressing down on your uterus every so often to make sure it's shrinking down as opposed to enlarging, which can be a sign of too much bleeding. If you have an epidural, you will feel nothing or just some pressure. Without an epidural, it can feel painful, so feel free to ask for some ibuprofen or Tylenol.

14. If you had an epidural, the catheter tip in your back will be removed. This usually doesn't feel like anything (yay!).

15. Eat, drink, and stare in wonder at the baby you just birthed! If you're wondering if they will always look the way they do right now (and it's OK if you have that thought), head to page 221, "Will they always look . . . like this?"

16. Some hospitals have you stay in the same room for your entire hospitalization, but others may have you transfer to a new room on

the postpartum unit. This is for all patients who've given birth, whether vaginally or by C-section. If you are moved to a new room, this usually happens a few hours after giving birth, after your team is done monitoring you closely. Page 235, "Who is around to help me figure all this out?," goes into this in more detail.

SHOULD I ASK FOR DELAYED CORD CLAMPING?

Yes! Though to be honest, in most places this is standard practice, since we know it's so beneficial for your baby, so there's no need for you to request it.

Delayed cord clamping means not placing an umbilical clamp until sixty seconds or more after birth. This generally tends to be the time that most hospitals will recommend, and it is also my personal practice (unless someone requests longer, which I am happy to do unless I have a medical concern).

When I was first in training, we used to clamp that cord almost immediately. The thought was that if we waited longer, the risk of bleeding would increase (which we now know is not the case). We also didn't think much of the benefits of delayed cord clamping. Thanks to better data and a recognition of what many midwives knew for a long time, delayed cord clamping is now the standard.

Fun fact: If cord clamping is delayed for just sixty seconds, an extra ⅓ cup of blood gets to baby!

Here's why we love delayed cord clamping:

	Which leads to . . .	Dr. Jen's notes
Gets more blood from the placenta to baby, which means more iron and red blood cells for baby	Lower rates of iron deficiency in the first twelve months of baby's life	Iron deficiency can lead to poorer motor and brain development.
	Less likely to need a blood transfusion	This is especially important for preterm infants, for whom these risks are significantly higher and can be fatal.
	Lower risk of necrotizing enterocolitis and bleeding in the brain	
Keeps baby attached longer	· Promotes skin-to-skin contact, since they are less likely to be quickly taken to a baby warmer and separated · Improves baby's transition to life on the outside	Any practice that supports the golden hour (page 219, "What is this 'golden hour' I keep hearing about?") is great for both mom and baby.

We do know that there is a small increased risk of jaundice in newborns who've had delayed cord clamping, but this is often mild and easily treated with phototherapy (a "bili blanket" or "bili lights"). It's not concerning enough for us to not offer delayed cord clamping, but if you have concerns, talk with your team.

I do want to bust a common myth that during delayed cord clamping your baby has to be held at a level below your placenta for it to work (meaning they can't be placed right on your belly). **This is not true,** so if you encounter that, feel free to let your team know that you want that baby on your abdomen or chest right away—even at the time of a C-section!

Lastly, there are some scenarios where delayed cord clamping just can't be done. If your baby needs help immediately, then your doctor or midwife will have to cut that cord to get them to the pediatric team. If you're bleeding too much or are otherwise medically unstable, the same may need to be done. Sometimes in these scenarios we can "milk" the cord to get some of that blood to baby in lieu of delayed cord clamping, so that is something you can certainly ask for.

SHOULD I BANK MY BABY'S CORD BLOOD?

"Cord blood" refers to your baby's blood that is in their umbilical cord. It's a topic of interest because it contains **stem cells,** which are cells that can differentiate and become a number of different types of cells. Why do they get so much attention? Because these cells have been used in some medical breakthrough treatments for cancers, immunologic disorders, and genetic disorders that might be otherwise hard to treat.

Here are the top facts I cover when answering this question:

1. **This isn't cheap.** If you go the private banking route (I'll describe the differences below), this can be expensive. They will charge fees for collection, processing, and yearly storage.
2. **Delayed cord clamping should be prioritized.** See the above section for why, and know that this can mean there might not be enough blood left over for cord blood banking.
3. **Routine banking is not recommended by leading medical organizations.** This is because the chance of you or a family member using the cord blood is extremely small (1 in 2,500). The one exception is if a family member (such as a sibling) has a condition where a cord blood transplant could help. In that case, you'll want to talk with your medical team and genetic counselors while you're still pregnant to discuss private banking.
4. **The blood from your baby can't be used to treat the baby.** If your baby has a genetic condition, their own cord blood stem cells will not work (because these cells will carry the same genetics).

5. **Ask about financial incentives.** If you see cord blood banking advertised in your doctor's office, ask if they are being paid to promote it. If kickbacks are involved, that needs to be made clear.

6. **Even if you plan to do it, it may not be possible.** Sometimes emergencies arise and we can't stop to collect this blood.

7. **Consider public banking.** I wish everyone could do this! Keep reading for more.

Two types of cord blood banks exist, and they are very different. I was lucky enough to donate the cord blood from my first birth to a public bank, and it felt awesome knowing we were potentially helping save a life.

	Public bank	**Private bank**
What it is	Banks that store cord blood that can then be matched for use through a national donor program, or for research purposes. Think of it like donating blood.	It uses a company's service to collect and store your cord blood, which you can then use in the future if need be.
Cost	Free	Collection fee ranges from $1,000 to $3,000 and annual storage fees range from $100 to $300 on average.
Is your cord blood reserved only for you?	No	Yes
Availability	Not available at all hospitals. The National Marrow Donor Program has a list of which hospitals are currently offering this: **https://www.nmdp.org/what-we-do/partnerships/global-transplant-network/cord-blood-banks-and-hospitals**.	You can order a kit to be sent to your house, so they are widely available.

	Public bank	Private bank
Benefits	• The ability to help people and advance lifesaving treatments! • No cost to you	You have access to your own cord blood if needed
Drawbacks	No access to your own cord blood in the future	• Very low likelihood of use • Cost

Whatever you decide, the important part is that you **let your team know ahead of time,** as public banking is not available everywhere (unfortunately!) and you'll often need screening bloodwork done in your pregnancy to qualify to donate to them if you are planning to go that route. And when it comes to private banking, you'll need to order your kit and bring it to the hospital when you are admitted—we don't stock these on Labor and Delivery.

WHEN (AND HOW) DOES THE PLACENTA COME OUT?

The placenta is the coolest organ in the body . . . and no, I am not biased. What other organ do you grow, that then grows another human, and once its job is done it gets the message to self-destruct and evict itself within a matter of minutes? Told you so. There's no competition.

The placenta is the star of the show of the **third stage of labor,** which is the time from when your baby arrives to when the placenta delivers. On average this takes just a few minutes, but it can take up to thirty minutes and still be considered normal. The feeling of the placenta coming out is like a sensation of pressure and then huge relief as it exits. It is a very different sensation from birthing a human, much to the relief of the person doing the birthing!

We know that performing some interventions can help your placenta come out and decrease your risk of bleeding too much or experiencing a postpartum hemorrhage. These include:

Intervention	Why we do it	Dr. Jen's notes
Giving medicine like Pitocin right after your baby is born	Helps the uterus contract, which helps the placenta to detach	Given as a shot or in your IV, this is recommended as routine in hospitals because we know it works very well at decreasing your risk of hemorrhage. You can decline it, but know this is one I really believe in.
Massaging the top of your uterus	Same as above	This can be painful if you don't have an epidural.
Immediate skin-to-skin contact with your baby	Increases oxytocin release, which is even better than synthetic Pitocin	Yet another reason to love skin-to-skin contact . . .
Applying gentle traction on the umbilical cord	Facilitates placental separation	"Gentle" is the key here. If done too aggressively, the cord can detach from the placenta. Your provider may then need to place a hand in the uterus to get the placenta out.

If your placenta is not coming out on its own, you may need something called a **manual extraction** for what is now called a **retained placenta.** This complicates about 1 to 3 percent of all pregnancies, so while it's not very common, it is something every OB-GYN and midwife has seen and managed.

A manual extraction is done by your provider placing their hand in your uterus to grasp and guide the placenta out. If you have an epidural, this will feel either like nothing or pressure like needing to have a bowel movement. If you don't have an epidural, your nurse can give you pain medicine in your IV to help. If that isn't enough, sedation, nitrous oxide, or general anesthesia is an option.

If this isn't successful, or if some of the placenta is still stuck (which we can see on ultrasound), you may need to go to the operating room for further treatment. There we can use more anesthesia if needed and potentially use tools such as suction or sharp curettage to remove the placental tissue. If the placenta is still not separating, this can be a sign of abnormal placental attachment, called **placenta accreta spectrum.** The treatment for this is often a hysterectomy.

But I want you to focus on the fact that most placentas—in all their awesomeness—often come out fine and in a matter of minutes!

SHOULD I TAKE MY PLACENTA HOME?

You've got options when it comes to your placenta:

	What it is	**Dr. Jen's notes**
Do nothing and your team will send it to medical waste	This is the default.	This costs nothing and is what most people who have hospital births do.
Have it sent to pathology or the lab for testing	This may be recommended by your team if it may help in diagnosing something for you or your baby (such as an abnormal placenta or infection).	This can be associated with a cost that insurance may or may not cover (and, sadly, your team will have no idea about what that cost is because healthcare is not transparent). This can be important for your baby or your next pregnancy planning, however.
Donate it to research	Some hospitals do research on placentas, or the cord blood and stem cells associated with them, to help with advancements in diagnosis and treatments.	Ask your team during your prenatal care if you're interested to see if this is available. Often you'll need to have some screening done before you give birth.

	What it is	Dr. Jen's notes
Take it home and plant it	Like it sounds—you take home your placenta and bury it under a tree or bush that you plant to commemorate your new addition.	I never did this, but I kind of wish I had!
Consume it in the form of smoothies or powders/pills	You take home your placenta and process it, or someone local does this for you. More below.	The CDC has issued guidance warning against this practice, as there is a risk of transmitting an infection to the baby.
Leave it attached to your baby until it falls off on its own (which can take 1–2 weeks)	Often called a lotus birth, this is a practice that many hospitals will counsel against given the risk for infection in your baby. Reasons for wanting this may include spiritual practices or the idea that it is more natural and less stressful for baby.	There are no safety studies on this, but the concern is that once the placenta and cord are birthed they no longer have blood flow. This means they are dead tissue that decays and is ripe for bacterial growth. Some people place salt, herbs, and oils on the placenta to decrease infection and improve the smell, but these are not proven to make this practice safer.

When it comes to consuming your placenta—either raw or in pill form—the claim behind it is that doing so can decrease your risk for postpartum depression/anxiety, improve your iron levels, and aid in your milk supply. My issues with these are the following:

1. There's no data to support any of this. In fact, one 2023 study of 6,000 new moms showed those who consumed their placenta actually had higher rates of postpartum depression; we aren't sure why.

2. It also doesn't make sense that consuming your placenta (which is filled with progesterone) helps your milk supply, since it is the

sudden decrease in progesterone in your system that triggers your body to start making milk.

3. If you have iron-deficiency anemia, foods or supplements rich in iron are easy to find.
4. Services that make placenta pills are often in someone's kitchen and are not held to any regulatory or sanitary standards.

As with any decision about your body, I believe that ultimately you get to decide—and that includes what you do with your placenta! If you are considering taking it home or leaving it attached to your baby, talk with your OB-GYN or midwife during your prenatal care to see how this plays out on Labor and Delivery. You'll often need to sign consents and bring your own containers to transport it home, and it's better to know the process long before your placenta shows up.

> One last thought: If you do choose to consume your placenta, please reconsider if you've had GBS or any other infection (including at birth), or if your baby is preterm or medically fragile.

WHAT HAPPENS IF I NEED STITCHES?

As I mentioned on page 200, "How do I prevent tearing?," tearing during vaginal birth is common. Sometimes these tears are small or don't bleed and don't require any repair, but if you do need stitches, here's what you can expect:

1. Your provider will test to see if you can feel anything. Often an epidural provides enough numbness, but if not or you've had no pain

medication, they can use a lidocaine injection to numb you, so you don't feel anything.

2. They will stitch up the laceration with suture that is absorbable. This means it will break down over a matter of weeks and you don't need to have any stitches removed. This often takes just a few minutes, but it can take longer if the tearing is more severe or in a hard-to-see area.

3. Sometimes we need an extra pair of hands to help, so your provider might call in an assistant. And if there is increased bleeding, too much pain, or a tear that is very hard to see or more severe, we may need to move to the operating room for a better repair.

4. Once all is done, ice is your best friend for the next twenty-four hours. Your nurse will keep you in good supply with pads that have ice in them.

5. Peeing can burn, and wiping can hurt! The best thing to do is not to wipe too hard but instead to dab gently and use a spray bottle (called a peri bottle) filled with warm water to clean up after going to the bathroom. Take these bottles home—they make great bath toys when your baby is older!

6. You'll also be given numbing spray that helps numb the area, since it can hurt or be sore while you heal. Use this as you need it, and definitely take it home too—it works great on cuts and burns.

7. Often the best pain medicine for this kind of pain will be Tylenol or ibuprofen, but if that's not cutting it, let your team know and they can give you something stronger.

If you've had a more difficult laceration, such as a third- or fourth-degree tear (see page 200, "How do I prevent tearing?"), your doctor or midwife will likely prescribe some stronger pain medicine, and will probably want to see you back sooner than the usual postpartum visit to make sure it's healing well.

Worried about the first poop after having your baby? Head to page 255, "I am terrified to poop."

WHAT IS THIS "GOLDEN HOUR" I KEEP HEARING ABOUT?

This refers to the first hour after birth, during which all efforts should be made not to separate the mom-baby couplet. Anything that needs to be done (such as checking vital signs or doing an initial brief physical exam on baby) should be done with the baby on their birthing parent's chest.

We give it such a lofty name because there is data to show that this is an important and sensitive period for newborn and maternal physiology alike. Having direct skin-to-skin contact in the golden hour has been associated with the following:

For the birthing parent	For baby
More likely to be exclusively breastfeeding on discharge	More stable vital signs (like temperature)
Longer duration of breastfeeding	More likely to have a successful first feed at the breast
Less breast pain and engorgement at three days postpartum	Better glucose levels
Less anxiety at three days postpartum	Less likely to cry!
Higher satisfaction with their birth experience	

If the golden hour were a pill, we would be prescribing it for everyone, given this data!

I do want to acknowledge the two following scenarios that you might encounter:

1. **You've had a C-section.** The golden hour can (and should) still be respected if you have a cesarean birth, but I know many hospitals still have work to do in getting there. Many of the studies that looked at the benefits of skin-to-skin contact in this golden hour also included situations where it was initiated more than ten minutes after birth, so I don't want you to stress or feel that you missed the boat if your baby was first brought to a warmer, dried off, examined, and then brought over to you. This still counts and is fantastic!

"IS SKIN-TO-SKIN SAFE IN THE OPERATING ROOM?"

I want you to know that *many* myths persist about skin-to-skin contact in the OR. You might hear that the OR is too cold for babies to do skin-to-skin, it's unsafe because the baby could fall, your anesthesia team can't monitor you safely with a baby on you, and "it's just not how we do it." All of these myths have been debunked by studies, as well as by the fact that it is routine in many hospitals without any problems—so why not yours? A great question to ask during your prenatal care . . .

2. **You or your baby are not medically stable and must be separated.** Sometimes birth doesn't go according to plan and skin-to-skin contact isn't possible in the first hour, or even the first day or days. If this is the case, I want you to know all is not lost and you can still give your baby all that they need. What matters is that you and your baby are safe and supported. Having a partner or family member do this skin-to-skin in that hour (if possible) can be a fantastic substitute if you're not able to.

So yes, I really am saying that if unnecessary things—such as weighing or doing footprints—can be delayed until after this first hour, they should be. Will it annoy your family? Maybe. But this isn't about appeasing the group chat!

QUESTIONS TO ASK YOUR TEAM:

1. Is skin-to-skin for the golden hour routine at your hospital?
2. If I need a C-section, does my baby leave the operating room? Or is skin-to-skin standard in the OR? If so, how quickly will they be brought to me?

For more questions to ask your doc, see the checklist on page 307.

WILL THEY ALWAYS LOOK . . . LIKE THIS?

You are *not* a bad parent if you're handed your newborn and you have this as an initial thought! The short answer is no—but there's a good reason they look the way they do at this moment.

Coming through the pelvis is *not* a straightforward journey. This means your baby might have:

- A coned head
- Uneven head swelling
- Facial swelling
- Facial bruising
- Ears that are folded up
- Scrapes on their face or head
- An enlarged vulva or scrotum

Most of these happen from the normal squeeze they get as they go through the pelvic bones and birth canal. The head especially is meant to change shape to fit, which is why there are spaces or "soft spots" between the skull bones that allow for this movement. Others, like an enlarged vulva, can be from the hormones of pregnancy, which resolve in the weeks after birth.

Depending on the length of your labor and the position of your baby, as well as if interventions like placing an internal heart rate monitor or using vacuum or forceps were needed, their appearance can vary. And keep in mind that C-section babies can also have all these changes too, especially if you were in labor prior to having your C-section.

I often joke with parents that if they are alarmed by their baby's appearance, they can always wait until the next day to send photos out—it is amazing what twelve or twenty-four hours will do!

CAN I HAVE AN IUD PLACED RIGHT AFTER I HAVE MY BABY?

You sure can.

This is called a **postplacental** or **immediate postpartum IUD insertion,** and it is what it sounds like: Within about ten minutes of your placenta coming out, we can place either a hormonal or nonhormonal IUD in your uterus using our hand or a long grasper that can feed the IUD into the uterus. This can be done after either a vaginal or cesarean birth.

Here are some things to consider about having this done:

Benefits	Risks or potential drawbacks
Immediate birth control	There is an increased risk of it falling out (expulsion) when placed immediately (10% to 27%) as opposed to waiting until your postpartum visit for placement (2% to 10%).

Benefits	Risks or potential drawbacks
No need for a follow-up appointment for this	Can't be placed if you have ongoing heavy bleeding or an infection in your uterus or bloodstream
If you have an epidural, you often don't feel anything	If not planned ahead of time, your doctor or midwife might have trouble getting the IUD quickly enough to place it (not all labor and delivery units will stock them).
No data to show it has any effect on your milk supply, unlike some other forms of hormonal birth control	If you're delivering at a Catholic hospital, they may not allow this (or any form of birth control). See page 27, "Does the religious affiliation of my hospital matter?"

You might think it seems silly to do this, given the higher expulsion rate I mentioned, but since up to 40 percent of American women don't make it to a postpartum visit, this can be an opportunity to get what you need before you leave the hospital and life gets crazy!

Ultimately, I think that having more options to make birth control accessible is always a good thing, so if this is something you might consider, ask your doctor or midwife at a prenatal visit if this is something they can do.

CAN YOU EXPLAIN WHY MY BABY GETS SHOTS AND EYE OINTMENT WHEN THEY'RE BORN?

I can, and once again I consulted the pediatrician in the family, Dr. Doug, for his expertise on why these are routine practices in the United States.

Vitamin K shot

Vitamin K is essential to forming blood clots. We normally get it from our food and our gut bacteria, but newborns strike out on both these fronts because breastmilk is very low in it and their gut can't make it yet. **All newborn babies are deficient in this important vitamin.** This is why it is a routine injection given within the first six hours of birth. Babies who do not receive this shot are at much higher risk of developing bleeding problems (this risk is almost zero if they get the shot)—and this risk lasts for a full six months after birth. Babies who bleed because they lack vitamin K will often hemorrhage in their brain, with 1 in 5 babies dying from it.

Vitamin K fast facts:

- Oral vitamin K does not work as well as the shot.
- You've never heard of a baby bleeding from a lack of vitamin K because you live in the United States—in other countries that don't routinely give the shot, it is more common.
- It does not cause cancer (this was based on an older, disproven study).
- It has a "black box" warning about severe allergic reactions, but these are almost all from giving the medicine differently (via an IV); only one case in a baby was ever recorded during decades of use.
- Most doctors will not clip a tongue tie or circumcise babies without this because they have an increased risk of bleeding.

Erythromycin eye ointment

Back in the day, some babies developed severe cases of conjunctivitis (pink eye), and some of those babies were blinded by the damage to the eye. Eventually we found out that it was caused mainly by the gonorrhea bacteria, and that it was preventable by putting a one-time smear of an antibiotic ointment called **erythromycin** on newborns' eyes. Thankfully, we now test and treat pregnant people for this STI, so the risk of this eye infection is lower, but not zero. Babies can also develop conjunctivitis from other bacteria, and the ointment lowers this risk as well.

Hepatitis B vaccine

Hepatitis B is a virus that damages the liver, and one of the problems with it is that most people don't know they have it until decades later, when the damage is done. Untreated, it can cause hepatitis, cancer, and liver failure. It is spread from mother to baby in the uterus as well as through blood, saliva, and sexual contact. It is *far* more infectious than HIV because an infected person's bloodstream can have about 100 times the amount of hepatitis virus than HIV virus.

You might be wondering, "I was tested for this in pregnancy and was negative, so why does my newborn need this vaccine?" (I had this *exact* question and resistance when I learned about this vaccine in my first pregnancy.)

Here's why:

1. Only half of hepatitis B infections occur from mom to baby in the uterus.
2. In the United States before the vaccine was introduced, around 10,000 children every year were infected from people other than their mother (for example, an infected family member *who doesn't know they have it* has a small cut on their finger, and that finger goes in your baby's mouth).
3. Hepatitis B is far worse when you get it as a child.
4. Thus, a vaccine at birth drastically reduces the chance your baby will get the virus.

One teaspoon of blood from someone infected with hepatitis B can have 5 billion infectious virus particles in it!

What if I have concerns about vaccines?

As I said earlier, some practices will not care for kids unless they are fully vaccinated. If you plan to not vaccinate your child or pursue a non-evidence-based vaccine schedule, you should clarify this prenatally so you aren't left without a doctor for your baby unexpectedly once they arrive.

If you want an evidence-based place to go for vaccine-related questions, Dr. Doug can't recommend this site highly enough: **https://www.chop.edu/vaccine-update-healthcare-professionals/resources/vaccine-and-vaccine-safety-related-qa-sheets**.

Dr. Doug also believes that children who are not fully vaccinated deserve access to high-quality healthcare, and thus he works hard to partner with families to make sure they feel heard, can communicate their concerns, and make a decision that is based on science, data, and trust—not on misinformation.

CAN THEY BATHE MY BABY BEFORE I HOLD THEM?

While we can do that, we actually recommend skipping the immediate bath. This means we generally put baby—gunk and all—right up on your belly or chest after they arrive. If that seems gross, keep reading. There is science behind it!

You might feel relaxed and pampered after a bath, but for a newborn they can actually be very stressful. We know that early bathing of newborns (defined as less than six hours old):

- Can cause hypothermia (low body temperature), even when warm wipes or water is used
- Can cause hypoglycemia (low blood sugar)
- Can interrupt skin-to-skin time
- Can lead to lower breastfeeding rates (likely because of separation and stress to baby)

We also know that babies come out covered in varying amounts of **vernix.** This is the white cheesy stuff that you may have heard of, and for good reason: It can help seal in moisture that protects your baby's skin, conveys scents to you that can help with bonding, and may also have antimicrobial properties.

The World Health Organization currently recommends delaying any newborn baths until twenty-four hours after birth. Many U.S. hospitals will wait at least eight hours, with some not doing any bathing prior to discharging you. There are some situations where a bath is recommended to decrease the risk of an infection like HIV or hepatitis going from uterus to baby, however.

My personal take is to delay that bath as long as possible for all the reasons mentioned above. That may mean no bath until you get home, and that's OK! You can spot clean with water and wipes in the groin area as needed. If your baby is covered in meconium, your team might recommend wiping that off or getting any gunk (scientific term) out of their hair, but you don't need to use soaps or cleansers or to get them pristine the moment they come out.

If the idea of a slippery, wet baby covered in amniotic fluid and blood freaks you out, it's OK to ask that your baby have a quick dry wipe before they're put on you. But if you can hold off on a full bath first thing, I think your baby will thank you for it!

THE AFTERPARTY

HAVING A BABY IS SO FUN!

You get to . . .

1. Grow your baby for ten months (sorry, 40 weeks is ten—not nine—months; please don't shoot the messenger).
2. Squeeze a watermelon out of your vagina or have major abdominal surgery while awake to birth said watermelon.
3. See your baby and think, "Wow, will they always looks like . . . *that*?"
4. On second thought, of course they look more like Dad, naturally. That feels really fair.
5. Immediately be the source of nutrition for a new human who knows literally nothing about feeding other than he must eat now and even though the nipple is *in his mouth* he is *freaking out* and, hello evolution, *why is this the best we've done?*
6. Wear your own diaper to remind you just how much of an adult you really aren't at this moment.
7. If you've had a C-section, have people cheer for you when you (1) stand up, (2) don't vomit, (3) finally fart.
8. Have your nipples on display when anyone tries to come visit, like your grandfather, the cafeteria guy, or the twelve-year-old med student . . .
9. . . . all while watching your partner with his useless nipples sleep on the couch that he tells everyone "isn't that comfortable."
10. Applaud yourself for not choosing violence for #9.
11. Fill out more paperwork than any sleep-deprived human should ever be legally allowed to do.
12. Be asked about birth control, as if you will *ever* have sex again (spoiler: you probably will).
13. Get discharged with your new human to drive on roads where everyone is clearly maniacal and out to get you.
14. Enter your home. Feel that no one has ever done this before and survived it all. But you will—just one hour at a time.

HOW LONG DO I STAY IN THE HOSPITAL FOR?

In the United States, people who have a vaginal birth usually stay in the hospital for one to two days after. For a cesarean birth it can range from two to four days.

Of course, this isn't always the case. I've had some patients who deliver vaginally go home twelve hours later, and others who need to stay longer if there are any concerns or complications regardless of how they gave birth.

The reality is that some new parents are ready to get out of the hospital ASAP, while others are terrified to leave. And those with other little ones at home see the time in the hospital as a vacation of sorts where you've got only one kiddo to look after (this was me with my second—I just loved having food brought to me—but eventually they kicked me out).

Regardless of how your baby made their appearance, here is what needs to be happening for your team to feel OK about sending you home:

1. Your pain is under good control with medicines you can take by mouth.
2. Your bleeding is in the normal range (like a period, give or take).
3. Your vital signs are normal and don't cause us to worry that you have an infection, lost too much blood, or have high blood pressure.
4. You can empty your bladder, and if you've had a C-section, you're passing gas (No need to poop before you go home! But if you're worried about that, see page 255, "I am terrified to poop").
5. Feeding your baby—however you choose—is going well.
6. Your baby's vital signs are normal and they're making good diapers (which reassures us about #5).

7. You've got a car seat that your baby fits into.
8. You have a plan for follow-up appointments for you and your baby.

WHERE DOES MY BABY STAY?

Once your baby arrives, one of these places will be their hospital home:

1. In your room with you 24/7.
2. In your room, but with a nursery they can be sent to if you request it.
3. In a separate nursery, brought to you when you request it.
4. In an intermediate nursery because of a minor medical concern.
5. In the neonatal intensive care unit.

For healthy newborns in the United States, the first two options tend to be the most common. Gone are the days of all babies being kept in a nursery where parents would have brief visiting hours and the babies would be put on display like an exhibit at the zoo (I mean, that *was* kind of weird, right?).

Most leading medical organizations, including the American Academy of Pediatrics, recommend fully rooming in with your baby as the preferred choice. This means that except for brief times when your baby may need to be taken out of the room for tests that may not be able to be performed in the room, they stay with you for a total of twenty-three to twenty-four hours a day.

Studies have looked at whether rooming in is good progress . . . or just plain exhausting for new parents.

Here's what's been found:

Benefits of rooming in	Possible drawbacks
Increased number of breastfeeding sessions, which can support milk supply establishment	May not get as good quality of sleep (but data is conflicting on this)
Lower amounts of formula supplement given	Can be hard if medical complications are impacting your recovery and your ability to care for your baby
Parents are better able to identify and respond to baby's hunger cues	Could increase the chances of unsafe bedsharing
Increases confidence in parenting skills because parents are more involved and can be supervised by nursing staff in their rooms	May feel harder for birthing parents who don't have a partner or other supporters with them
May help some parents sleep better, as they know their baby is there with them	Some hospitals that do rooming in have done away with any kind of respite nursery, which can make getting help a challenge if your nurse is busy with many patients, if you need to go to the ICU or OR, or if you have other complications
Allows for family-centered care, as parents are present for all baby examinations and most tests	
Allows for baby to be held by you during vaccinations or blood tests, which has been shown to decrease pain in newborns	
Safer from a security standpoint	

It's important to know what to expect, so I recommend that you ask your doctor or midwife how your hospital's postpartum unit works during your pregnancy. It's not ideal to think you'll be getting eight hours of undisturbed sleep while your baby is in a well-baby nursery only to show up and learn that rooming in is the only option. This can also give you the chance to decide to give birth in a place that has the arrangement that feels right for you.

I do want you to know that rooming in doesn't mean you're left to fend for yourself. Keep reading to see who will be there to be by your side.

WHO IS AROUND TO HELP ME FIGURE ALL THIS OUT?

Can you believe you just made a human and now you must keep it alive—sometimes after just having had a major abdominal surgery, or having your vagina stitched up? Yeah, it's OK to have a WTF moment and wonder how you're going to do all this. The good news is that you're not in this alone.

While the exact look of your postpartum team may vary by hospital, this is the support you can generally expect:

1. **Your labor and delivery nurse.** They are usually with you for a few hours after your delivery and are crucial in ensuring that you and your baby are off to a good start. They can help with your baby's first feed, your immediate pain control, your bottom's icing, and your first bathroom trip.

2. **Postpartum nurses.** As I mentioned on page 206, "What happens when the baby comes out?," most hospitals have separate postpartum units where you'll go for the remainder of your stay after your baby arrives. Many hospitals provide couplet care, which means the same nurse cares for you and your baby (IMO, this is best: You and your baby are one dyad, so this just makes sense). Your nurse's job is to make sure you and your baby are healthy and have everything you need—things like pain medication, monitoring for your bleeding, and assistance with the hardest part no one talks about, which is swaddling your baby. I'm kind of joking, but also not (swaddling memories make me sweat). Your nurse will also make sure your baby is doing well by monitoring their vital signs and ensuring they have all their needed tests completed (like monitoring for jaundice and a hearing check) before discharge. They're also usually the first person to help with breastfeeding, and many have specialty training in this. But if they aren't, or if you need more help, that brings me to . . .

3. **The lactation consultants.** I have so much more about breastfeeding in the coming pages, but you should know that lactation consultants can be a critical part of your breastfeeding journey. Keep reading to learn more about them and how to get their help.

4. **Certified nursing assistants.** Also called CNAs, these are often the people who will take your vital signs, get supplies, help you with walking after a C-section, get you clean bedding, do newborn hearing screens, weigh your baby, help set up your breast pump, get formula or donor milk, provide emotional support . . . the list goes on! Think of them as a critical helper to your postpartum nurse.

5. **Your obstetric team.** Once you have your baby, we don't disappear! Your provider (or those covering for them in the hospital) will see you daily to make sure you are recovering well, or more frequently if there are any concerns. Your postpartum nurse stays in communication with them if any issues arise. If you have a question for them outside of these visits, your nurse can page them if need be.

6. **Your pediatric team.** This may be your baby's pediatrician or a partner in the practice covering for them, or it may be a hospital-based pediatrician or nurse practitioner who will see your baby daily. This is something you can ask about if you do a meet-and-greet visit with a potential pediatrician; I describe this more on page 40, "When should I pick a pediatrician?" They'll do a full exam when they first see your baby and a more targeted exam daily until discharge. Tip: Write down all your questions to ask them when they stop by, so you don't forget when you're so focused on watching your baby get their first check-up!

7. **Housekeeping.** Hospital housekeepers are angels who keep the unit running.

8. **Nutrition services.** Often our favorite folks, they bring you your meals (and often enjoy sneaking a peek at a cute baby).

The reality of healthcare these days is that with the focus on profits and cost savings, many hospital administrators have cut back on clinical staffing. This means your nurses and doctors are often doing more with less. I am saying this not to scare you but to let you know that if you feel you aren't getting the help you need from the folks above, please speak up and let us know. We want to give you the best care, and sometimes the higher-ups need to hear from patients to know what didn't meet the mark so that they can move some of that money from their end-of-year bonus to actually helping people.

WHAT DO I DO FOR PAIN?

It's important to know that pain after having a baby is normal, no matter how you gave birth. Your body just went through a major event, and recovery takes time. The good news is that we've got lots of options to help ease the way, so let's cover those.

Be aware that usually you'll have to ask for medication, as it won't be automatically brought to you. If you find this bothersome and are worried you will forget and fall behind on pain control, ask for your medications to be scheduled. This means your nurse will get an alert when they are due rather than relying on you to ask for them. You can always decline taking them, but I usually order my patients' medications this way so that they don't have to worry about keeping track of another thing when they're tired and recovering.

When it comes to narcotics (opioids), though, these tend to be reserved for pain not controlled by our other options. They do have a role in recovery—so don't feel guilty if you need to use them—but given their risk of addiction, we understandably want to make sure we are using them correctly and only when needed. If you take narcotics at baseline for chronic pain issues, let your team know that you likely will need higher doses and will need a good pain plan so that your needs are met.

I want to reassure you that all these medications are safe for breastfeeding, even narcotics, with one caveat: We do know that narcotics containing codeine or tramadol can be riskier. They can cause excessive sleepiness or breathing problems in newborns whose breastfeeding parent takes them. This is because up to 5 percent of Americans are ultrarapid metabolizers, which means more of the drug ends up in breastmilk.

For this reason, I'd personally recommend starting with oxycodone if a narcotic is needed and **avoiding Tylenol with codeine (Tylenol #3) or tramadol (Ultram).**

Here's what you can have available postpartum:

Medication	What it is	Dr. Jen's notes
Ibuprofen	An anti-inflammatory that works great for uterine cramping after birth	This is my go-to for all postpartum patients who can have them.
Acetaminophen (Tylenol)	A pain reliever that works well for mild to moderate pain	This can be given with ibuprofen together, or in an alternating schedule.
Ketorolac (Toradol)	Think of it as an injectable version of ibuprofen	This is often given if you're having a C-section in case you're having nausea and might throw up pills.
Narcotics like oxycodone (when Tylenol is added to oxycodone, the combination is called Percocet), **hydrocodone (Vicodin), codeine** (when combined with Tylenol, it is called Tylenol #3), or **hydromorphone (Dilaudid)**	Opioid medications work well for more severe pain; they will usually be given in pill form but also come in injectable forms if needed	We try to avoid these in routine vaginal births, but sometimes they are needed if the above medications aren't enough. These are often used for pain after a C-section, but many patients do well without them, as we are getting better at using other treatment methods. Avoiding codeine and tramadol is generally recommended if you're breastfeeding.

Medication	What it is	Dr. Jen's notes
Numbing sprays (such as Dermoplast)	A topical benzocaine that numbs the skin	We often use this after all vaginal births. You can spray it on after you pee or as needed. Also great for hemorrhoids.
Numbing patches (such as a lidocaine patch)	A patch that can be placed near a painful area, such as a C-section incision	These can be great to try if you've had a C-section, but their use isn't routine yet. You can ask for them!

Let's also not forget about ways to treat pain that don't come in a bottle:

- **Heating pads.** These can be great to help with uterine cramping or soreness elsewhere, like your back.
- **Ice.** As I mentioned on page 217, "What happens if I need stitches?," it's your best friend for the first twenty-four hours after a vaginal birth. You can use it longer too, so just ask if you need more.
- **An abdominal binder.** This can be helpful after having a C-section, but I do want to stress that this isn't meant to be worn 24/7. It can give some nice core support when you are up and about, but also know that overuse can actually weaken your muscles over the long term since you aren't relying on them as much. Your incision also should be open to the air most of the time for healing, too. Lastly, this is *not* meant to "train your waist" or help with whatever Instagram is trying to sell you in this moment!
- **Walking.** Walking to *treat* pain? I know it might sound strange, but walking is *so* important to help wake up your bowels and move that gas through, especially after a C-section. Gas pain can be way worse than any incisional pain, so yes, I want you cruising around in your room and in the halls! It also helps get any extra fluid back into circulation, so that you can pee it out. This can be really great if you had preeclampsia or got super swollen during the labor process.

- **Relaxation techniques.** I am not here to pretend that meditating is going to fix all your pain, but I do want to acknowledge that these techniques can work in conjunction with other interventions.

Before I wrap this up, I need to acknowledge that Black and brown women are often undertreated when it comes to pain (yes, there's data to back this up). If you feel you aren't being taken seriously, head to page 138, "I don't feel I'm being listened to. What are my options?," for ways to get the treatment you need and deserve. But if this happened to you, I am sorry and I want you to know we are working hard to improve the care you deserve in this country.

HOW DO I BREASTFEED?

It's the most natural thing in the world—you just put baby to breast, and it works.

"Ha ha," said anyone who has ever breastfed—myself included!

The best way to learn how to breastfeed is . . . to do it. It's like riding a bike in that we can explain how it works and make sure you know where to put your feet and find the brakes, but nothing can replace the actual experience.

But this doesn't mean you can't prepare and know some guidelines, so with that I give you my top ten tips for getting breastfeeding off to a decent start:

1. **Prepare long before your baby pops out.** "But, Dr. Jen, you just told me . . ." I know. What I mean is that prepping is good, but nothing replaces on-the-job training. I can't recommend in-person lactation classes enough. Ask your doctor or midwife what they recommend, as many hospitals run their own, or a community lactation consultant may offer them. This gives you the chance to get hands-on practice, ask questions, check out a pump and learn how to use

it, and maybe even identify a lactation consultant who you can have on speed-dial if needed once you give birth. Virtual classes or even online programs are an option too, as is reading a good breastfeeding book, so figure out what might work for you.

2. **Know the reality that is breastfeeding.** And the reality is that, yes, breastfeeding is "natural," but so are hurricanes. That doesn't mean it's always easy to navigate, and that doesn't mean you're doing it wrong. The first time you tried to walk, you didn't just get up and do it, right? The same goes for you and your baby, who are learning together. It's OK for it to not be perfect and to stumble! Which leads me to . . .

3. **Know the warning signs of when you might need help.** If any of these happen, it's time to ask for some extra assistance:

   - You have pain that is not getting better.
   - You aren't able to get your baby to latch, or to stay latched.
   - Your baby is inconsolable at the breast.
   - Your baby is not feeding enough based on their age or diaper output.
   - You're about to lose your shit.

4. **It *can* be uncomfortable.** Especially in that first week or two, the pain of your baby latching can be intense. I remember dreading it and my toes curling when it happened. This pain is normal if it only lasts for a few seconds but then goes away. If it doesn't go away, this can be a sign that the latch is not right; if this isn't addressed, it can cause severe damage to your nipples. Unlatch that baby and ring your call button for help!

5. **Maximize skin-to-skin contact.** If skin-to-skin contact were a drug we could prescribe, we wouldn't be able to keep it in stock. Data shows that skin-to-skin in the first hour after birth (but also in those first days, too) can make breastfeeding more successful. For more on this, head to page 219, "What is this 'golden hour' I keep hearing about?"

6. **Watch your baby, not the clock.** You'll often hear guidelines that your baby should feed every two to three hours, for a total of eight to twelve feeds in twenty-four hours, and that each feed should last ten to fifteen minutes on each side. Cool. But babies can't tell time. Sometimes they want to feed a whole lot more frequently (called **cluster feeding**) and then zonk out for a stretch of four to five hours. Sometimes they want to chill at your breast longer because it's their happy place. Don't feel guilty feeding your baby more and responding to their cues—in fact, please do respond to their cues! Think of those guidelines as minimums and ask your team for other ways to know your baby is getting enough.

7. **Minimize visitors.** Having too many visitors who want to see you and hold your baby can mean you might miss feeding cues, your baby may get fussy and then be a mess when it comes time to eat, or you may feel too embarrassed to nurse in front of your grandfather. It's OK to say no to visitors during your postpartum stay, to limit them, or to cut their visits short.

8. **Don't view supplementation as a failure.** Sometimes babies need more milk than our boobs can make at that moment in time. In these scenarios, supplementation—either by donor breastmilk, or by formula—can be lifesaving. I am referring not to a topping-off-your-baby-because-it-can't-hurt supplementation but rather to medically indicated supplementation for reasons such as excessive weight loss or being preterm. I want you to know that in these scenarios, supplementation that is thoughtful and evidence-based can actually protect the breastfeeding relationship and be a key in its success. Please don't think you are a failure if this is needed.

9. **Know who is available in the hospital to help you—and use them!** I cover this in the next section, but know that you are not bothering us when asking for help. If you're told you don't "need" to see the lactation consultant but you want to, inform your nurse that you still want to and ask how that request will be communicated.

10. **Focus on you.** You can't care for another human if you don't care for you. Your only job during your postpartum stay is to feed yourself, feed your baby, and rest. And maybe walk a bit to help with recovery—but other than that, let it go. We don't need fancy thank-you bags, your friends don't need social media updates, and your family doesn't need to be entertained. You've got this.

MY FAVE PLACES TO GET TIPS FOR BREASTFEEDING

La Leche League USA

KellyMom: Parenting and breastfeeding support

Stanford Medicine Newborn Nursery: Getting started with breastfeeding (fantastic videos on hand expression, well-fed-baby checklist, and more)

National Women's Health and Breastfeeding Helpline: Free help with breastfeeding or other health issues (in English and Spanish), 9 A.M. to 6 P.M. EST, Monday through Friday, at 1-800-994-9662

InfantRisk Center hotline: Free call center staffed with experts about questions regarding medications and breastfeeding, Monday through Friday, 8 A.M. to 3 P.M. CST, at 1-806-352-2519

MommyMeds app: From the Texas Tech University Health Sciences Center's InfantRisk Center, this app has up-to-date information about prescription and over-the-counter medications and their safety during pregnancy and breastfeeding

Breastmilk storage tips from the CDC

Going back to work tips from WIC Breastfeeding Support

WHO CAN HELP ME WITH BREASTFEEDING?

Not all breastfeeding assistance is created equal. And some hospitals have policies where only people having problems get seen by the lactation consultant, usually because of staffing issues. This can make it difficult to see the lactation consultant if you need help—so speak up if you feel you aren't being heard.

Also, the term "lactation consultant" doesn't always mean the same thing—it could mean either an international board-certified lactation consultant (IBCLC) or a certified lactation consultant (CLC), who can have vastly different amounts of training and experience. Keep in mind, not every hospital has all these folks available 24/7, if at all. This is a great thing to clarify during your pregnancy!

Keep reading to decipher who can help you while you're in the hospital:

Type of support	Their training	Dr. Jen's notes
Your nurse	Most labor and delivery and postpartum nurses have some breastfeeding education requirements, though the quality and amount can vary.	This is often the first person to ask for breastfeeding help. Note that many nurses also have additional training and may also be an IBCLC. If you feel you need more help than they're providing, it's OK to ask that they call the lactation consultant.

Type of support	Their training	Dr. Jen's notes
International board-certified lactation consultant (IBCLC)	This is the highest degree for breastfeeding education. Certification includes: • 90 hours of lactation-specific education • College-level health science courses • 300 to 1,000+ clinical practice hours • Passing a certifying exam • Ongoing maintenance of certification	These are the pros in the breastfeeding world! They may not be available nights, weekends, or holidays, so ask your nurse about their availability if you want to see one.
Certified lactation consultant (CLC) **Certified breastfeeding specialist (CBS)** **Certified breastfeeding educator (CBE)**	The names vary, but think of these as a stepping-stone to becoming an IBCLC. They require: • 20 to 120 hours of classroom training • Often passing a written exam or completing a certification process offered by the training organization	These folks can offer great support, but for more complicated care an IBCLC is ideal.
Peer support (La Leche League Leader, WIC peer counselor)	Requirements can include: • 18–50 hours of classroom training • Personal breastfeeding experience	These are often not found in hospitals but can be great community resources once you go home.
Your doctor, midwife, or your baby's doctor	Most OB-GYN, family medicine, and pediatric training programs provide some level of breastfeeding education, but it is *highly* variable.	I won't lie—unless they've taken a personal interest in breastfeeding, many doctors don't have nearly enough training. Some (like myself!) have gone on to also become an IBCLC. It's OK to ask that they arrange a consult with the lactation specialist if you need more help than they are giving you.

FIND AN IBCLC

For help finding an IBCLC in your community, search the International Lactation Consultant Association's Find a Lactation Consultant Directory.

I DON'T WANT TO BREASTFEED, SO WHAT SHOULD I DO?

The first thing you should do is let go of any guilt, though I know this might be easier said than done.

I am a huge supporter of breastfeeding: I nursed my two kids, I went on to become an IBCLC, and I was the medical director of a breastfeeding clinic. But all this actually taught me that while breastfeeding can be amazing, it definitely isn't free, it doesn't always work out, and we need to make sure all new parents are supported and not made to feel guilty if they are unable to or choose not to pursue it for any reason.

Here are my dos and don'ts if breastfeeding isn't part of your plan:

DO:

- **Confirm that this is an informed decision** and not because people or social media have scared you off breastfeeding. Chat with your doctor, midwife, pediatrician, and support network. Once you're sure, keep reading.
- **Consider where you give birth.** You may have heard of the term "baby-friendly hospital"—these are hospitals where the staff and policies reflect a culture of breastfeeding support. I think these can be amazing, but if you're not planning to breastfeed, delivering at

one of these might make your decision feel like an uphill battle (though not always, I promise!), and you may want to consider not delivering at a baby-friendly-designated facility.

- **Make sure your team knows your plan** and ask that they document it in your chart.
- **Communicate this verbally** once you are on Labor and Delivery, and make it clear you don't want to be asked over and over again about it.
- **Consider putting a sign on your door** that says "Formula feeding" or "Donor milk feeding" so that, again, you won't get asked repeatedly.
- **Ask for a lactation consultant to see you.** See a lactation consultant when you *don't* want to breastfeed? Yes! Even if you aren't nursing, your postpartum body may need some support, as hormones in the early days often have other plans. An IBCLC can help you with support; they are experts in helping people wean!
- **Wear a well-fitted bra** that is supportive but not too tight.
- **Use cool compresses** to help relieve breast pain or swelling.
- **Take ibuprofen** to help with pain and inflammation.
- **Express just a little milk** to soften your breasts and make you comfortable if your breasts feel engorged or painful when your milk comes in.
- **You can ask about drugs to prevent your milk from coming in, but know that these aren't commonly used.** One, called **cabergoline,** has data showing that it works and is well tolerated, but it's not FDA-approved for this specific use in the United States quite yet (though it can be prescribed off-label). A single dose of **Sudafed** (the version containing pseudoephedrine) can also decrease milk supply, but it should be avoided if you have high blood pressure, as it can make this worse. Sometimes multiple doses are needed.
- **Consider using chilled green cabbage leaves,** as some data shows this can help reduce inflammation (but other studies show no effect, so don't worry if you can't get your hands on it).

DON'T:

- **Breastfeed in the hospital only because you've been guilted and shamed into it.**
- **Bind your breasts.** This is advice that I hope is becoming less common, but I still hear it now and again. Doing this can cause the ducts in your breasts to clog, which can lead to mastitis. Some cultural practices support this, so if you choose to do it, be mindful of signs of plugged ducts and mastitis so that you can seek help if needed.
- **Take birth control with estrogen in the first three weeks** (and potentially longer—more on this on page 257, "What is the birth control situation?"). You may read about this helping to suppress milk supply, but in the first three weeks it can increase your risk of life-threatening blood clots.
- **Use heat packs on your breasts.** This can cause more swelling and inflammation.
- **Rely on herbs too much.** While herbs such as peppermint and sage are often said to decrease milk supply, there isn't great data to support this (though to be clear, the risk of a few Altoids a day is almost nonexistent!). If you're considering using them, your IBCLC can help guide you with information so that you can make an informed decision.
- **Feel you can't change your mind.** If you decide after a few days you do want to breastfeed, ask your team for guidance.

SHOULD I DO VAGINAL SEEDING IF I'VE HAD A C-SECTION?

I hesitated about putting this question in the book because I feel like it was a big thing on social media a few years ago and then seemed to fizzle out. But I eventually decided to cover it because stuff tends to resurface and there's a lot of potential for misinformation with this one.

Vaginal seeding is the practice of intentionally wiping some of your vaginal secretions on your baby's skin, nose, and/or mouth to expose them to the bacteria they may have "missed out" on being exposed to because they were born by C-section. The theory behind it is that it helps your baby get exposure to your bacteria, which then colonizes their gut. This, in theory, decreases their chance of developing issues like asthma and other immune disorders that we see in higher numbers in babies born via C-section.

In general, we do *not* recommend this practice for the following reasons:

1. **Your baby can be exposed in other safer ways.** Breastfeeding and coming in contact with your breasts accounts for 40 percent of your newborn's microbiome! In other words, a huge amount of the good bacteria your baby can get from you has nothing to do with your vagina.
2. **We haven't proven that being born by C-section increases risks of certain disorders.** It is true some studies have shown increased asthma risks in C-section babies, but it's likely much more complicated and includes environmental and genetic factors as well.
3. **Any differences in newborn gut microbiomes disappear by six months of age.** So it's hard to say a short-term difference causes diagnoses later in life that would justify vaginal seeding.
4. **It hasn't been proven to be safe.** We lack studies that tell us babies who've had vaginal seeding don't get sick more than babies who haven't had this done.
5. **There's a real risk of infection.** We can't say that swiping vaginal secretions directly into your baby's nose or mouth is the same as it happening in labor, when there are multiple other hormonal and chemical factors related to the process of labor at play. This could

potentially increase the risk of your baby getting an infection and becoming rather ill.

Because of the above, major medical organizations do not recommend vaginal seeding outside of scientific studies. And if through those we do learn more and it appears to be safe, you can guarantee I'll be the first to let you know!

If after reading this you still want to proceed, **please reconsider if your baby is preterm or you are GBS positive, had an infection in labor, have genital herpes, or have other infectious diagnoses like HIV.** These can pose huge risks to your baby. If your baby becomes ill and this was done, please also let your child's pediatrician know so they can do an appropriate workup.

WHAT DO I NEED TO KNOW ABOUT TONGUE TIE?

In the briefest of nutshells:

1. Tongue tie is real.
2. It can cause issues with breastfeeding.
3. Breastfeeding problems are rarely based on one thing.
4. Tongue tie can be overdiagnosed. It can also be underdiagnosed.
5. It's important to be evaluated by a knowledgeable breastfeeding provider if you are having any difficulties or not meeting your feeding goals.
6. If your pediatric provider brushes off tongue tie as a "fad," you may want to seek additional lactation help from someone else.

Tongue tie, officially known as **ankyloglossia,** is when the tongue is restricted because of an abnormal attachment to the floor of the mouth via a band of tissue called the **sublingual frenulum.** We all have this attachment, but when it's too far forward or too short, it can restrict how well the tongue moves up and out.

In combination with *many* other factors—nipple shape and size, how high a baby's palate is, muscle tone or tightness, other medical issues with mom or baby—this can impact feeding from the breast and the bottle. It can result in painful breastfeeding, poor milk transfer and poor milk supply, and a very frustrated parent and baby.

If I want you to remember one thing, it's that **tongue tie is a functional diagnosis.** That means it cannot be diagnosed just by looking. What matters is how the tongue moves and functions during the process of feeding.

That said, not all tongue ties cause breastfeeding problems. Also, the same frenulum and tongue may not be causing any issues in the first few days but might do so later as your milk supply changes. This is why it's essential that you have a discussion with someone trained and knowledgeable in breastfeeding—ideally an IBCLC—who can do a detailed assessment.

If tongue tie appears to be impacting breastfeeding, management can include:

1. **Lactation support** to try different positions and techniques to improve latch.
2. **Assessment of your baby's jaw and neck muscles.** If these are tight or not allowing for a proper latch, fixing this through massage or gentle bodywork can help. Sometimes this is all that is needed.
3. **Using a nipple shield** to help your baby latch better and protect your nipples. The goal is not for this to be a long-term fix, as it may cause milk supply issues over the long term, but it can be a helpful bridge as your baby grows and their suck improves. An IBCLC can

help you decide how best to size one and make sure your care plan is supportive of your long-term goals.

4. **Frenotomy,** a quick and simple surgical treatment where the band of tight tissue is cut to restore normal movement to the tongue. After numbing gel is placed, your baby is swaddled and the thin restrictive tissue under the tongue is visualized and released (it's not actually the tongue muscle itself). The actual release of the tongue tie takes only a few seconds. This often costs a few hundred dollars and is almost always covered by insurance, but you can ask ahead of time to confirm.

A *lot* of misinformation exists about frenotomies, so I want you to know that:

1. There is no difference between using scissors and using a dental laser for this procedure in newborns. The important part is the comfort and skill of the provider doing it.
2. Risks are rare and include bleeding and infection.
3. Reasons to not have it done include not having been evaluated by a lactation consultant first and increased risks of bleeding in your baby (such as if there's a family history of bleeding disorders or if they've not had their vitamin K shot—more on page 223, "Can you explain why my baby gets shots and eye ointment when they're born?").
4. To achieve the best outcomes, the tissue needs to be released completely. This means that if only part of the restrictive band is snipped, it may help some, but if it doesn't, your baby may need a second procedure to fully get the outcome you were hoping for.
5. Numbing medicine can be used on gauze before the release for pain control.
6. There is disagreement about the importance of post-procedure wound management. The mouth heals quickly, and sometimes the

two edges of the snip under the tongue can heal back down together and create a restriction again. Evidence around how to best care for the incision site is limited, so discuss options with your provider and IBCLC.

7. Exercises to move the tongue, jaw, neck, and to help your baby get more comfortable with latching and positions after a tongue-tie release are important and should be directed by your provider and/or lactation consultant.

WHAT'S UP WITH CIRCUMCISION, AND WHO DO I ASK?

Circumcision is a cosmetic decision, not a medical one. Either your pediatrician or your OB-GYN can be the go-to for this procedure. They may perform the circumcision in the hospital before your baby goes home, or have you come into their clinic in the first few weeks after discharge to have this done (where it often costs less).

This is an elective procedure, so if your baby is preterm, has health concerns, or isn't feeding well, or if your doctors are unable to get to it because of other responsibilities in the hospital, then it will be delayed and may not happen before you go home.

Aside from religious or cultural reasons, the following are commonly cited reasons one might want their baby circumcised, along with my thoughts:

Potential benefit	Dr. Jen's notes
Fewer urinary tract infections (UTIs) in the first twelve months	About 111 circumcisions need to be performed to prevent one UTI (which are very rare in boys, and easily treatable with antibiotics).

Potential benefit	Dr. Jen's notes
Slightly lower risk of sexually transmitted infections	Can be reduced better by safe sex practices like condom use and vaccination.
Lower rates of penile cancer	Very rare: About 300,000 circumcisions would need to be done to prevent one case of cancer. This is also preventable with HPV vaccination.
Prevents the possibility of the foreskin becoming too tight or stuck (phimosis)	This can usually be treated with topical cream if it happens. Circumcision to treat it is not often needed.
Potentially easier for hygiene	Regular cleaning with or without foreskin is easy for boys to learn.

I think you can tell from my notes where I stand with circumcision, and I really come at this from a lens of bodily autonomy. I've also heard parents say they want their child to feel "normal" in a locker room or in a relationship—and I think it's important to reflect on how and if we teach our children whether paying attention to others' opinions of their genitals is acceptable or not. You might think I am getting too deep, but I believe it's important to take a high-level view here.

Rates of circumcision are decreasing in U.S. hospitals: In 1978, 65 percent of babies were circumcised, and this rate dropped to 55 percent in 2016. Overall, about 70 percent of men in the United States are circumcised, according to 2016 data. There are definite regional variations too, with the lowest percentages of boys being circumcised in the West and the highest percentages in the Midwest.

Lastly, while some potential benefits are there, they are small and not without risk, such as scarring, infection, bleeding, and decreased penile sensation during masturbation and intercourse (though, overall, physical complications are rare, at about 0.4 percent).

I am aware that there are some traditions that support circumcision, but I do want to end this section by calling to attention some of the ethics of this practice:

1. Is it ethical to perform a cosmetic procedure on a minor who can't consent?
2. Is it ethical for us to continue to do male circumcision when female circumcision has been determined to be unethical?
3. Is it more ethical to delay such a procedure until the person is older and can decide for themselves?

I AM TERRIFIED TO POOP.

I know. I was too after I had my babies. The idea of straining and potentially tearing any stitches, or using your belly muscles after having a C-section, can almost seem scarier than the birth itself. But there are things you can try to make it better!

Here are my tips on making that first bowel movement more comfortable:

NON-MEDICATION INTERVENTIONS		
	How it works	**Dr. Jen's notes**
Minimize opioids (narcotics)	These cause constipation, so using other medications for pain control can prevent this.	Sometimes you need to take them, and that's OK! Just try to limit your dose and use some of these other methods below.
Stay hydrated	This can help prevent constipation and hard stools.	Drink enough until your pee is pale yellow.
Walk	Walking helps things move through, which is extra important if you've had a C-section.	Take it slow and steady, but get those steps in.

<table>
<tr><th colspan="3">NON-MEDICATION INTERVENTIONS</th></tr>
<tr><td>Chew gum</td><td>If you've had a C-section, this can help your bowels "wake up" sooner and decrease time to passing gas and your first BM.</td><td>The data isn't great, but it's a low-risk "intervention."</td></tr>
<tr><td>Eat fiber-rich foods</td><td>Think prunes, kiwi, mango: These draw water into the bowels, softening your poop.</td><td>Good evidence these can help, and few side effects.</td></tr>
<tr><th colspan="3">MEDICATIONS</th></tr>
<tr><td></td><td>How it works</td><td>Dr. Jen's notes</td></tr>
<tr><td>Docusate (Colace)</td><td>Advertised as a stool softener, but there is little evidence this works at all.</td><td>Skip it! Ask for something that works better.</td></tr>
<tr><td>Psyllium (Metamucil)</td><td>Soluble fiber that bulks the stool and draws water in.</td><td>Safe and few side effects.</td></tr>
<tr><td>Polyethylene glycol (Miralax, GoLYTLEY)</td><td rowspan="2">Laxative that softens the stool by drawing in water.</td><td rowspan="4">· Good evidence these all work.
· Safe for short-term use.
· May cause diarrhea and cramping.</td></tr>
<tr><td>Magnesium oxide</td></tr>
<tr><td>Senna (Senokot)</td><td rowspan="2">Stimulates the bowels to contract.</td></tr>
<tr><td>Bisacodyl (Dulcolax)</td></tr>
</table>

Despite there being almost no evidence Colace works—and that there is known harm in avoiding giving other medications first that could prevent constipation better—many hospitals still have it as the go-to on their orders (mine included). If you are prescribed this, don't hesitate to ask for something better from the table above, such as Senokot (my personal fave, and I promise they didn't pay me to say that).

Let me also say that if you've had a C-section, it's very likely that you won't poop before you leave the hospital. As long as you are passing gas, that's totally normal and tells us things are moving through fine. You'll probably have your first BM the first day or so home, but if you're feeling backed up you can add one of the medications above or consider using an enema.

WHAT IS THE BIRTH CONTROL SITUATION?

If you're not wanting to get pregnant right away and are having sex with someone who produces sperm, you need a birth control plan. We generally recommend not putting anything in your vagina for four to six weeks (though I cover how there isn't much data to support this on page 260, "I forgot all the discharge instructions so . . . can you repeat them?"), but the reality is that **up to half of all people who give birth have vaginal sex before six weeks postpartum**—so we gotta talk contraception!

There are *lots* of options out there, but I want to highlight these three super-important facts:

1. **No estrogen-containing birth control before twenty-one days postpartum**—and potentially longer if you have certain risk factors. This is because the risk of blood clots is too high.
2. **There is no one-size-fits-all approach.** The best method is the one that feels right for you.
3. **Depending on the religious affiliation of your hospital, your doctor or midwife may not be able to use or prescribe some of these methods.** More on this on page 27, "Does the religious affiliation of my hospital matter?"

Here's a quick overview on different options:

Method	Pregnancy rates in 100 people using this method for 1 year	Dr. Jen's notes
Abstinence	0	Great if it is acceptable to you and your partner
Arm implant (Nexplanon)	Less than 1	• Can be placed in the hospital before you leave or at your postpartum visit • Limited data shows no decrease in your milk supply if placed before discharge (as opposed to waiting for six weeks postpartum)
IUD	Less than 1	Can be placed right after birth (see page 222, "Can I have an IUD placed right after I have my baby?") or at your postpartum visit
Tubal ligation	Less than 1	• Can be done immediately postpartum or as a separate outpatient procedure • Only do this if you are 100% sure you are done having kids!
Vasectomy	Less than 1	• Takes three months (to wash out the sperm already in the reproductive tract) before it can be relied on for birth control • Only do this if you are 100% sure you are done having kids!
Birth control shot (Depo)	6	• Can be given before you leave the hospital if you want it • Theoretical risk it may decrease your milk supply if given in the first forty-eight hours, but there's not much data to support this concern • Requires a shot every three months
Lactational amenorrhea	2–8	• Must meet strict criteria to rely on this method (baby is less than six months old, periods haven't returned, exclusively or nearly exclusively breastfeeding, pumping doesn't count)

Method	Pregnancy rates in 100 people using this method for 1 year	Dr. Jen's notes
Estrogen-containing methods **• Combination pills (estrogen + progestin)** **• Vaginal ring** **• Patch**	9	• Avoid in the first three weeks postpartum (blood clot risk) • Avoid up to six weeks postpartum if you are at high risk for blood clots • If you are breastfeeding, consider waiting until breastfeeding is well established (four to six weeks) to prevent the possibility of estrogen decreasing your milk supply (there isn't great data about this, but worth weighing the risk/benefit to unplanned pregnancy)
Mini pill (progestin only)	9	• Needs to be taken within the same three-hour window every day to work (Slynd is one exception in this group and has a twenty-four-hour window) • Same theoretical risk on milk supply as the shot, with limited and conflicting data
Condoms **Diaphragms** **Cervical caps**	12–24	• Some diaphragms require an office visit to fit you for the right size • Requires 100% compliance to work
Withdrawal	22	Requires depending on a partner and full compliance
Fertility awareness method	24	• Often called "natural family planning" • Requires a lot of effort (tracking your temperature, cervical mucus, symptoms, etc.) but certainly can be doable if you're committed • The FDA-cleared app Natural Cycles can be used to make this easier and more reliable
Spermicide	28	Best used in combination with another method

This is *a lot* to review in your postpartum sleep-deprived haze, so in a perfect world you've discussed this with your doctor or midwife ahead of time at your prenatal visits. But if not, don't stress: There's always time to decide what's right for you as long as you aren't having vaginal intercourse in the meantime.

> My absolute favorite resource to get more information on these methods and do side-by-side comparisons is **Bedsider.org**.

I FORGOT ALL THE DISCHARGE INSTRUCTIONS SO . . . CAN YOU REPEAT THEM?

You bet. Between all the paperwork, follow-up appointments, and going home with an actual human you must care for, leaving the hospital can be overwhelming. It's very normal if your eyes glazed over when your provider or nurse was reviewing your discharge instructions.

Let me say these three things up front:

1. Don't leave the hospital until you have a phone number you can call 24/7 for both you *and* your baby in case you have urgent questions.
2. Postpartum healing takes a while, but in general each day should be about the same or better than the one before. If you feel like you're going backward, please let us know.
3. I break down when to get in touch with your doctor or midwife on the following pages, but if something feels like an emergency and it's not on the list, or if you don't think it can wait, get the care you need ASAP. You know you and your baby best.

WHEN TO CALL 911 OR GO TO AN EMERGENCY DEPARTMENT

- Bleeding enough that makes you feel lightheaded or you pass out
- Intrusive thoughts about harming yourself or your baby
- Your partner notices unusual behavior in you, like hallucinations
- Chest pain
- Shortness of breath
- Uneven leg swelling that may or may not also be red or tender
- The worst headache of your life
- Seizures or possible seizure-like activity
- Signs of a stroke: slurred speech, uneven facial appearance, one arm or leg not working
- Sudden vision changes like not being able to see out of one eye
- Your partner has hurt or threatens to hurt you or your baby

WHEN TO CALL YOUR DOCTOR OR MIDWIFE **NOW**

- Bleeding that soaks a pad in one hour for two hours straight, or clots larger than an egg
- Pain that is not well controlled by the medications we've sent you home with or is suddenly worse or increasing
- Temperature of 100.4 degrees F (38.0 degrees C) or higher
- A headache that doesn't get better with Tylenol or ibuprofen
- You can't keep anything down
- If you've had a C-section and have any redness, hardness, or drainage from or around your incision
- If you had a vaginal tear and felt a popping sensation around your stitches, or have sudden pain in the area

WHEN TO CALL YOUR DOCTOR OR MIDWIFE **FIRST THING IN THE MORNING**

- Feeling that mentally you're having more bad days than good days
- Breastfeeding issues such as:
  - Redness or streaking that could indicate mastitis
  - Hard lumpy areas that don't drain with feeds
  - Nipple pain that lasts the entire feed, or any signs of nipple damage
  - Any concerns that breastfeeding is not going well
- Vaginal discharge that has you concerned about an infection
- Signs of a bladder infection (pain with peeing, foul-smelling urine, feeling like you have to pee all the time only to pee small amounts)

REASONS TO CALL YOUR PEDIATRICIAN

- Your baby's rectal temperature is 100.4 degrees F (38.0 degrees C) or higher
- Any concerns with feeding
- Fewer diapers than expected (should be one wet diaper for every day old—i.e., four wet diapers on day four, and by one week old and beyond should have six to eight wet diapers every twenty-four hours)
- Poops that are watery like diarrhea, go back to being black and sticky, or have any visible blood in them
- Projectile vomiting (not just spitting up)
- Dark-colored pee or any concerns about color or smell (note: reddish crystals in the first few days are normal)

- Any yellow or green eye discharge
- Umbilical cord or circumcision site concerns: bright red bleeding, odor, redness
- Your baby is super irritable or won't stop crying
- Jaundice (yellower skin and eyes) that is worse
- Your baby is very sleepy and hard to wake up
- Your baby doesn't seem to be breathing right (such as the skin between their ribs sucks in when they breathe, or they are breathing fast and hard)
- If anything doesn't feel right or you have any questions

GENERAL DISCHARGE INSTRUCTIONS

1. **Pain.** Continue your pain medication that you've been using in the hospital as you need. You can often taper after a few days. It's also OK to keep using heat and ice as needed. Soft pillows to sit on can help if you've had a vaginal tear or painful hemorrhoids.
2. **Constipation.** Do your best to avoid it! See page 255, "I am terrified to poop," for more on what to use. If you've had a third- or fourth-degree laceration, definitely make sure you've got a good bowel regimen and avoid using any medicines in your rectum to prevent disrupting those stitches unless cleared by your provider.
3. **Bleeding.** This is normal up to six weeks postpartum but should decrease over time. It may increase when you get up after lying flat for a few hours, or with an increase in activity. It's also normal for it to change color from bright red to darker red to brown and even black the further out from your delivery you get. We usually recommend pads over tampons, to decrease your infection risk, but there's not great data here, so it's up to you. It can be a good idea to avoid tampons if you've had stitches, however, since they could get stuck on the threads and hurt.

4. **Activity.** The most important thing is to listen to your body and to not push yourself beyond what feels right for you. You can get back to exercising whenever it feels right—just start slowly and stop if you have an increase in bleeding or too much pain. There are no rules on avoiding activity like running or lifting weights after a routine vaginal birth, but if you aren't sure if something is OK, just ask. I talk more about what to do after a C-section below.

5. **Vaginal sex.** There's no data that says you must wait for any specific amount of time to have sex safely. There's a theoretical risk of increased infection when the cervix is still open a little and bacteria could get into the uterus more easily, but we don't have studies to support that, and we also don't tell people they can't have sex when they're on their period, which is another time when their cervix is open a little. Yet this is dogma that has been repeated over and over again, so we seem to have come to believe it's based in fact. That said, you can choose to wait until your postpartum visit to ensure you've physically healed, or you can have sex sooner if it feels comfortable for you. Go slow, use lube if needed, and stop if it hurts. Don't forget the birth control if you don't want to get pregnant! And if you've had more severe tearing, ask your doctor when it is OK to resume sex, since that can take a bit longer to heal. **When to have sex is also entirely your choice, and whether or not you've been "cleared" for sex doesn't mean you need to have it.**

6. **Healing your vagina.** You can continue the care you've done in the hospital, and if you're having pain or swelling with a vaginal tear, you can consider sitz baths (submerging your vulva in warm shallow water—do not add anything with fragrance!—for a few minutes a few times a day; kits are sold to make this easy to do) for relief. But what about a nice warm soak in the tub? . . .

7. **Tub baths.** We often tell people not to take a bath until four to six weeks after birth because of a theoretical risk of infection. However (once again . . .), there is no data to support this. It's probably

not a bad idea to avoid hot tubs and pools, as more bacteria can live in them, and to not soak in water if you've had a C-section until the skin has healed, but beyond that, it's up to you.

8. **Incontinence.** Let your provider know if you are leaking urine, gas, or poop. A little bit of urine or gas leakage can be normal in the immediate postpartum period, but we definitely don't want to miss something more than this that can impact your quality of life but is treatable. Which leads me to . . .
9. **Healing your pelvic floor.** Consider requesting a referral to a pelvic floor physical therapist. These are specially trained physical therapists who help manage pelvic floor disorders, and we know that birth—whether vaginal or by C-section—affects your core and pelvic floor. In France, all women get a referral to them after birth . . . isn't that nice? I'd definitely recommend this if you had a vacuum or forceps birth, had a third- or fourth-degree laceration, had a big baby, or pushed for three or more hours.
10. **Hemorrhoids.** These are very common and can hurt and bleed. You can try sitz baths (data shows that adding Epsom salts to warm water can make this pretty effective), over-the-counter numbing creams, and ramping up the bowel regimen so you don't have to strain. Call your provider if you are in severe pain from them, as they may need to be treated with a procedure like banding or removal.
11. **Mood changes.** The baby blues are very common and normal, but signs of postpartum depression or anxiety should *not* be ignored. Read below for more on this as well as postpartum psychosis, which is a true medical emergency.
12. **Breastfeeding.** See above for when to reach out to your team, but also ask for recommendations for local lactation consultants who your providers recommend, in case you need them. And check out the other sections on breastfeeding in this book for more info!
13. **Birth control.** If you're not using any birth control method, you can get pregnant just a few weeks after having a baby! Make a plan that

feels right for you (see page 257, "What is the birth control situation?"), or if there's a slip-up, consider **emergency contraception** (in the form of morning-after pills like over-the-counter Plan B or the prescription ella, or the copper IUD) if you don't want to be pregnant. Head to Bedsider.org for more information on these and how to pick the best one for you.

IF YOU WERE DIAGNOSED WITH PREECLAMPSIA:

- Don't leave the hospital until you have a blood pressure cuff to monitor yourself at home (and know how to use it) and you've scheduled an appointment to have a blood pressure check (no later than ten days postpartum, but ideally sooner).
- You are still at risk postpartum, including for **postpartum preeclampsia.** See the boxes on page 268 for warning signs and how to get care, which can be lifesaving.
- Check your blood pressure as your team directs you or at least twice a day. See the box for reasons to alert your team.
- Continue any blood pressure medication as instructed. Call if you feel dizzy after taking it or notice that your blood pressure is dropping lower than normal—these can be signs it's time to lower your dose or stop your medicine. But don't do this without checking with your provider first!
- Lifelong, if you were diagnosed with preeclampsia, you are twice as likely to have heart disease and five times as likely to develop high blood pressure. It is *essential* that your primary care providers (for the rest of your life!) know of this diagnosis, as this changes how they'll screen for these across your lifespan. The document "My Health Beyond Pregnancy" is a great tool to communicate your risk and track your health (you can find it in the Resources section, page 297).
- Be sure in any future pregnancies that your providers know your history. Since you are at higher risk for developing preeclampsia again, they'll want to discuss ways to lower that risk.

SAVE YOUR LIFE:

Get Care for These POST-BIRTH Warning Signs

Most women and postpartum people who give birth recover without problems. **But anyone can have a complication for up to one year after birth.** Learning to recognize these POST-BIRTH warning signs and knowing what to do can save your life.

Trust your instincts. ALWAYS get medical care if you are not feeling well or have questions or concerns.

Call 911 if you have:	❑ **P**ain in chest ❑ **O**bstructed breathing or shortness of breath ❑ **S**eizures ❑ **T**houghts of hurting yourself or someone else
Call your healthcare provider if you have: (you only need one sign) (If you can't reach your healthcare provider, call 911 or go to an emergency room)	❑ **B**leeding, soaking through one pad/hour, or blood clots, the size of an egg or bigger ❑ **I**ncision that is not healing ❑ **R**ed or swollen leg, that is painful or warm to touch ❑ **T**emperature of 100.4°F or higher or 96.8°F or lower ❑ **H**eadache that does not get better, even after taking medicine, or bad headache with vision changes

Tell 911 or your healthcare provider:

"I gave birth on __________ and
(Date)
I am having __________."
(Specific warning signs)

Scan here to download this handout in multiple languages.

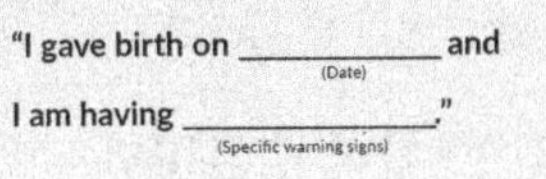

These post-birth warning signs can become life-threatening if you don't receive medical care right away because:

- **Pain in chest, obstructed breathing, or shortness of breath** (trouble catching your breath) may mean you have a blood clot in your lung or a heart problem
- **Seizures** may mean you have a condition called eclampsia
- **Thoughts or feelings of wanting to hurt yourself or someone else** may mean you have postpartum depression
- **Bleeding (heavy)**, soaking more than one pad in an hour, or passing an egg-sized clot or bigger may mean you have an obstetric hemorrhage
- **Incision that is not healing, increased redness, or any pus** from episiotomy, vaginal tear, or C-section site may mean an infection
- **Redness, swelling, warmth, or pain** in the calf area of your leg may mean you have a blood clot
- **Temperature of 100.4°F or higher or 96.8°F or lower**, bad-smelling vaginal blood, or discharge may mean you have an infection.
- **Headache (very painful), vision changes, or pain in the upper right area of your belly** may mean you have high blood pressure or post-birth preeclampsia

AWHONN
PROMOTING THE HEALTH OF WOMEN AND NEWBORNS

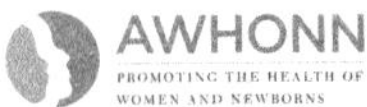

This program is supported by funding from Merck through Merck for Mothers. Merck for Mothers is known as MSD for Mothers outside the United States and Canada.

AWHONN thanks Kenvue for commercial support of the translations of this handout.

 16005

IF YOU'VE HAD A CESAREAN SECTION:

- **Wound care.** These are my top tips, and I think they are all super important:
  - Don't go overboard on your incision with scrubbing—all you need to do is let soap and water wash over it in the shower, and then pat it dry.

You are STILL AT RISK after your baby is born!

Postpartum Preeclampsia

What is it?

Postpartum preeclampsia is a serious disease related to high blood pressure. It can happen to anyone who has just had a baby **up to six weeks after the baby is born.**

Risks to You

- Seizures
- Stroke
- Organ damage
- Death

Warning Signs

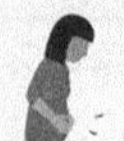
Stomach pain

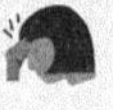
Severe headaches

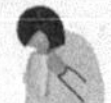
Feeling nauseous or throwing up

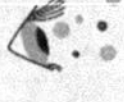
Seeing spots (or other vision changes)

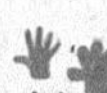
Swelling in your hands and face

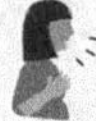
Shortness of breath

What can you do?

- Ask if you should follow up with your doctor within one week of discharge.
- Keep all follow-up appointments.
- Trust your instincts.
- Watch for warning signs. If you notice any, call your doctor. If you can't reach your doctor, call 911 or go directly to an emergency room and report you have been pregnant.

PREECLAMPSIA™ FOUNDATION

For more information, go to www.stillatrisk.org

After delivery - recognizing these signs can save your life

Call your healthcare provider right away If you can't reach your healthcare provider, call 911 or go to an emergency department and report that you have recently been pregnant.	• Blood pressure at or exceeding 140/90 • Severe headache that won't go away • Vision changes • Stomach pain • Swelling in your hands and face • Feeling nauseous or throwing up
Have someone take you to the ER or call 911	• Blood pressure at or exceeding 160/110 • Shortness of breath or trouble breathing • Seeing spots • Seizures

PREECLAMPSIA™ FOUNDATION

www.stillatrisk.org

- Stay away from scar creams or any ointments until *after* your skin is healed and your doctor has examined you.
- If your incision is in a skin fold that gets moist, it is important to make sure it's open to air frequently. Lie back, lift the skin, and then pat it dry, or use a hair dryer on the cool setting as needed. You can also use a fragrance-free pad or panty liner in the fold to wick away moisture, but this must be changed frequently so that it doesn't become a bacterial breeding ground.
- Check on your incision once or twice a day (or have a support person do it) to make sure it doesn't have any concerning signs, which are . . .
- If you see any redness, fluid or pus drainage, or separation, or if the area around the incision feels hard, snap a picture and call us. These could be signs of infection. Bonus points if you draw a line around any red areas so that we can track if it's spreading or improving over time.
- If you've been sent home with Steri-Strips (little white bandages) on your incision, these should be removed once your baby is seven days old. If left on longer, they can get crusty and icky. They may also fall off sooner than that, and that's totally normal. Getting them wet and then peeling them off makes removal easier.

- **Activity and lifting.** In addition to what I mentioned above, when you've had a C-section there are some extra guardrails. Most women are told after a C-section to not lift anything heavier than their baby and to not drive for six weeks. **There is no data to support these recommendations,** and frankly, these are unrealistic for most new parents (especially ones with older kids). So here's my advice, which takes into account the real world we live in:

    - Don't drive until you are off narcotics, can slam on the brake pedal, and can turn your head quickly. This timing will be different for different people. Cruise around the block first to practice before hitting the highway.

- When bending or lifting, use your knees—don't bend over and make your abdominal muscles do more work. A good place to start with lifting is to lift your baby. If that feels OK, put them in the car seat and try lifting the car seat. If it hurts, stop and only lift what you can without pain. Ask your adorable toddler to join you on the couch rather than picking them up when they ask. Bribe if needed—this is about survival. You've got this.

WHAT DO I DO IF I THINK I HAVE POSTPARTUM DEPRESSION OR ANXIETY?

Suicide and Crisis Lifeline: Call 988 (24 hours a day, 7 days a week, 365 days a year) or go to **https://988lifeline.org**.

Get help at Postpartum Support International: **www.postpartum.net**.

You should let your doctor or midwife know ASAP so we can help. There is no shame in experiencing this or seeking help for it—for you or your partner (yes, partners can get it too and have often been ignored when we talk about postpartum mood disorders).

In fact, **death by suicide or overdose related to these disorders is the leading cause of perinatal death in the United States.** Not hemorrhage. Not infection.

So we need to talk about it.

As I mentioned above, mood changes after giving birth are common—you're experiencing fragmented sleep and your hormones are rapidly shifting, all while you're trying to learn about your newborn and keep them safe and happy.

Here's what you need to know about what you (or your partner) might experience postpartum:

	Stats	What it is	How we treat it	Dr. Jen's notes
Baby blues	Affects 85% of birthing people	• First one to two weeks postpartum • Mood swings that can include crying, anger, irritability, but these are mild and limited	• Trying to get a stretch of four hours of uninterrupted sleep • Getting outside • Eating regularly • Usually resolves on its own	If you are crying at random commercials a few days after having your baby (like I was . . .), this is probably to blame!
Postpartum depression (PPD)	1 in 7, but may actually be higher	• Usually after two weeks postpartum • Depression • Fatigue • Hopelessness • Lack of connection to your baby	• Same as above • Antidepressant and/or antianxiety medications • Therapy	• We use standardized screening tools to diagnose these. They can even be given during pregnancy, since sometimes it can start then. • Our treatments work *really* well (but medications can take a few weeks). Many medications are safe in breastfeeding.
Postpartum anxiety (PPA)		• Anxiety symptoms (heart racing, sweating, racing thoughts) • Constant worry about your baby that sticks and makes you uncomfortable • Panic attacks		
Postpartum psychosis	1–2 per 1,000 people	• Hallucinations • Hearing voices • Lack of insight that these are not real • Thoughts of harming yourself or your baby	• True medical emergency • Admission to the hospital • Psychiatry consultation and medications	This can be really scary to witness as a partner, but it's so important to get care ASAP.

Note: All of these can be diagnosed up to twelve months after giving birth.

It's important to know that there are risk factors that make these diagnoses more likely. If you have a preexisting mental health diagnosis, experienced one of these in a prior pregnancy, have a family history of any of these, or have had a traumatic birth, you should be on high alert. Making a plan ahead of time with your medical team and your support network can make a huge difference in how your postpartum recovery goes.

I want you to know that it won't always be this hard, and that you taking care of yourself is so important. The world is so much better with you in it.

I THINK I HAD A TRAUMATIC BIRTH AND I DON'T KNOW WHERE TO GO FOR HELP.

> One in three people report their birth as being traumatic.
>
> One in five birthing people in the United States experience obstetric violence during their pregnancy and birth. That increases to one in three for BIPOC folks.

Let me be clear that this is not a weird question. You might be thinking, "Isn't it obvious if a birth was traumatic? Like a baby that had severe complications, or you ended up in the ICU, right?" Sure, that could qualify, but here are some other examples of what someone might identify as birth trauma:

- Labor going so fast you couldn't get an epidural, and you had an unplanned unmedicated birth.

- Poorly controlled pain despite trying medications or interventions.
- Feeling like your care team didn't adequately listen or address your concerns.
- The doctor you thought would deliver your baby was out sick and a stranger was there instead.
- You delivered preterm. Everyone is fine, but you were not ready for anything that happened.
- You ended up having a C-section.
- You wanted to do everything "all natural" but needed Pitocin and an epidural.

The point here is that birth trauma is subjective, and it doesn't have to be dramatic to "count." In fact, something like "just" needing a C-section might have rocked your emotional well-being and sent you to a dark place—but it's hard to get anyone to understand you because they all think it's no big deal.

And what about **obstetric violence**? This is the term for when someone is disrespected, treated without dignity, or abused by a person or system during the birth process in a way that causes them to lose their autonomy. Think cervical exams done without consent, using coercive tactics to get someone to agree to a C-section, or forcing someone to birth on their back when they clearly don't want to.

This term might sound startling, but I think it captures just how harmful this kind of treatment is. It also acknowledges that an act can be violence without being physical. Some OB-GYNs dislike this term and think the term "obstetric mistreatment" is more appropriate. This OB-GYN thinks that in the United States—the developed country that boasts the worst maternal outcomes and terrible racial disparities—we need not water down the words of the human rights violation that is not having a dignified birth experience. If you've had a traumatic birth, experienced obstetric violence, or just don't know but something isn't sitting right with you, I encourage you to speak up and get support. I cover this in some detail on page 176, "I had a traumatic birth before and I want to know how to have a better experience this time," so I recommend checking out that section to see who to talk to or how to talk about it.

You may want to:

1. **Schedule a visit with your doctor or midwife solely to debrief your labor and birth experience** (this can even be virtual if going back to that facility is triggering). Write down your questions and bring a support person. If they were involved in your trauma and that doesn't feel safe, you can reach out to Labor and Delivery to see if you could debrief with your labor nurse. You can also ask to have a patient advocate (employed by the hospital/clinic) to be present at any conversations if you think this may help.
2. **Partner with a therapist who specializes in birth trauma** to walk through and process what happened.
3. **Give yourself permission to grieve** that your birth didn't go as planned, rather than focusing on what you "should" be feeling in this moment.
4. **Seek out peer support,** either through local groups or online. (Just be mindful of the potential for internet rabbit holes. Check in with yourself after you've been on Reddit for an hour: Do you feel lighter or heavier?)
5. Some of my favorite **online resources** include:
    - **Make Birth Better:** UK-based group with excellent informational PDFs
    - **Postpartum Support International:** Has resources and free online support groups, including a BIPOC birth trauma group
    - **Birth Trauma Association:** UK-based group with amazing amounts of information

I hope this information will allow you to see that you are far from alone, and—if you plan to get pregnant again—to know that there are doctors and midwives out there who will take any past trauma into account and work hard to help you have a healing, respectful birth.

IS EVERYTHING NORMAL DOWN THERE? BECAUSE IT DOESN'T FEEL THAT WAY . . .

Earlier I mentioned routine discharge instructions when it comes to the care of your bottom and pelvic floor (page 260, "I forgot all the discharge instructions so . . . can you repeat them?"), but I want to make sure the following is loud and clear and give it its own section.

If any of the following is bothering you weeks to months (or years!) after having a baby, we want to know about it:

1. You have leakage of urine, gas, or poop.
2. You feel or see a bulge in your vagina or rectum (often called **prolapse**).
3. You need to put a finger in your vagina to help get all the poop out of your rectum.
4. Sex hurts.
5. You feel like you must go to the bathroom far too often, you barely make it to the bathroom in time, or you leak on the way.

These can all be signs of **pelvic floor disorders** that can be the result of having a baby, and sometimes they don't show up for years or progressively worsen over time. Risks are higher with multiple vaginal births, having a large baby, or having a forceps- or vacuum-assisted birth, but these disorders can also happen to anyone with a vagina.

Your OB-GYN can be a great first person to see for this, and they can do a physical exam to see what might be going on. They may refer you to a **pelvic floor physical therapist** and/or a **urogynecologist** (an OB-GYN with additional specialty training in the care of pelvic floor disorders) for further evaluation and treatment.

Potential treatments may include targeted physical therapy, pelvic exercises, medicine, bladder support tools, surgery, or a combination of several of these to get you the quality of life you deserve.

> Less than half of all women who leak urine regularly tell a doctor about it, so they suffer in silence. Let us know so we can help!

STILLBIRTH

THE REALITY OF LABOR AND DELIVERY

Everyone thinks Labor and Delivery must be a fun place to work—and there's no doubt it can be. But the hardest part of my job involves two things: being the person who ruins another person's life by telling them their baby is no longer alive, and then having to leave that room to be part of a birthday celebration for a joyful new family with a smile on my face.

In both scenarios, none of it is really about me at all. But it weighs on me as I carry these families from the former situation with me, wondering how they're doing now, or if they've gone on to have a better outcome since we last crossed paths.

I think about that moment suspended in air that will divide a couple's life into the "before" and the "after"—when, after searching for a flicker on the ultrasound screen, I have to turn to them and say, "I'm so sorry, but there is no heartbeat."

The guttural screams, or wailing, or complete silence, or a moment of eye contact with a whispered, "I knew it"—they're all normal responses that all of us in this scenario have witnessed.

I can't unsee or unhear them, nor do I think those of us who do this job should. We are so lucky to be the ones to walk this journey with you, even though it's a journey no one would have chosen.

Please know that we think of you often.

I don't want you to have to read this section. I am so sorry you need to. I do hope, though, that it can be at least a little helpful as you endure this moment.

You are not alone. About 23,000 babies are born still every year in the United States. This is about 1 out of every 160 babies. I share that number only to show you that there are others who have walked this path, who can potentially offer insight and support, and who can understand your grief, anger, or whatever it is you are feeling now and in the days and years to come.

I want to share that those of us who work on Labor and Delivery are unfortunately very experienced in caring for patients who have lost a baby. We are ready to do all we can to get you through this. I do think, however, that sometimes the best information comes from hearing directly from those who have experienced it. This is why I've listed resources on page 291, "Where do I go from here?," and I encourage you to check those out if you want more information.

There is no right or wrong way to feel right now. I hope these pages can help.

WHAT HAPPENS NOW?

If you have gone right to this question, please consider going back and reading the introduction to this section to ground you as you go through these pages.

If you've been told that your baby's heart has stopped beating—whether on an ultrasound if you came in for decreased fetal movement or after waking up from an emergency C-section where your baby did not survive—it is absolutely OK to fall apart, to scream, to tell everyone to leave, to sob, and to feel numb.

You can ask to be told what the next steps are, or you can ask to be left alone until you are ready to hear it. I am going to answer this question from the standpoint of you wanting to know what the next steps are after being told your baby has died before you've given birth:

1. Sometimes we may need to order an additional ultrasound or have another doctor come to your room to repeat the ultrasound to make the official diagnosis. It might seem like diagnosing a loss is always very clear, but because of ultrasound image quality it isn't

always straightforward. Some hospitals also require this in order to avoid any tragic mistakes. You may find this extra step comforting (to be absolutely sure), or feel that it prolongs the inevitable. Talk to your doctor about it if you have concerns.

2. Depending on other circumstances, we may recommend delivery now versus waiting until you feel ready. For example, if you have severe preeclampsia (which can be very harmful to your health) we are going to strongly suggest you not leave the hospital and that we work on helping you have your baby. But if you came in for decreased fetal movement and this diagnosis was made with nothing else being medically wrong, it can be an option to go home and schedule an induction or a surgical procedure after you've had some time. I describe more about delivery options in the pages to come.

3. We will offer whatever supports we have to you. This can include bringing in someone like a chaplain from our hospital spiritual care team if you want that, or having our social worker come talk to you to discuss how to have this conversation with other children you may have (more on this later).

4. If you're staying in the hospital, we may offer to move you to another room that isn't in the middle of Labor and Delivery so that you aren't hearing other babies being born. This isn't always an option, though, and for that I am sorry. It's also OK if you don't want to be moved.

5. We'll also do our very best to make sure others know what's going on, from the nurses to the housekeepers and folks who bring your food. We don't want them to come in and congratulate you on your baby when they don't know the scenario. We usually do this by noting it in your chart and putting a sign on your door.

6. We are going to ask you questions about your wishes, ranging from whether you want to see your baby and what medical workup you are interested in pursuing to whether you want burial or cremation.

This is *a lot,* and I tell my patients there are no right or wrong answers, that it's OK if you need me to repeat things multiple times, and that it's also perfectly fine to change your mind. I do want to note that we often do this at the beginning of any induction so that you have time to consider your options and not wait until the emotional moments after your baby is born. But it's OK to tell us to stop and that you'll let us know when you are ready to talk about these things.

7. We will then start your induction of labor or make arrangements for a surgical procedure called a dilation and evacuation. I have more about this in the next section.

WHAT ARE MY OPTIONS FOR DELIVERY?

Three main options exist: an **induction of labor,** a surgical procedure called a **dilation and evacuation (D&E),** and waiting for labor to start on its own. Not all hospitals are able to offer D&Es, as not all OB-GYNs are trained to do them. Most states with abortion bans will be unable to offer this procedure, and many Catholic hospitals also usually have limited doctors on staff who routinely do these, so this can affect the availability of this option.

That said, if you have the choice, it's important to know that all these options are safe (though waiting for labor to start naturally may not always be recommended as I describe below) and are a truly personal decision. Knowing the details can help:

	What it is	Benefits	Drawbacks	Dr. Jen's notes
Induction of labor	Inducing labor in the same way as for a live birth	• You can see and hold your baby after delivery if you want to • Having a vaginal birth may be meaningful for some people • If you choose autopsy, the results will be more accurate	• Can be a long process • Labor pain • Higher rates of complications when done earlier in pregnancy, such as in the second trimester (i.e., infection, needing a D&C to remove the placenta, bleeding)	• This can often be started right away, or if you are medically stable you can go home and come back in a few days when you feel ready. • If you don't want to feel any pain, you can ask for an epidural even before the induction starts. • Needing a D&C to remove a stuck placenta is more common earlier in pregnancy.
Dilation and evacuation (D&E)	A procedure where the baby and placenta are removed through the cervix using surgical tools. This can be done in a hospital or in an outpatient clinic or surgical center.	• Quicker • You can be asleep for the procedure • Lower risk of infection or hemorrhage when compared to an induction	• Not all OB-GYNs or hospitals offer these • Procedural risks include uterine perforation, injury to the cervix, bleeding, and infection • Usually a multi-day process, as the cervix needs time to dilate via the use of medicine or laminaria • The baby is not intact after the procedure, so autopsy and holding may be limited	These are extremely safe procedures overall.

	What it is	Benefits	Drawbacks	Dr. Jen's notes
Waiting for natural labor	Allowing labor to start on its own	• May feel less medicalized and more natural • Allows you time to go home, process, and prepare your support network	• Can prolong the process and increase anxiety • Theoretical risk of blood clotting problems due to carrying a demised baby are uncommon, but increase the longer you wait (10% by four weeks) • Depending on how long you wait, this can affect how your baby looks once they are born and the ability to do genetic testing	• About 75% of people will go into labor within two weeks. • This is not a safe option if there are medical concerns for you.

WHAT ABOUT A C-SECTION?

We usually try to avoid this major surgery in the setting of a loss. However, in some scenarios we might consider it if your chances of uterine rupture are very high if we tried to induce labor, or if this is strongly preferred. Discussing this thoroughly with your team, including what this might mean for any possible future pregnancies, is key.

WHAT CAUSED THIS?

While every stillbirth has a cause, we can't always make a diagnosis. These can be the hardest losses because it not only leaves you without answers but also can make it hard to know what to do in your next pregnancy to not have this happen again.

We know some of the causes of stillbirth, which in the medical definition includes any loss after 20 weeks gestation:

Cause	Frequency	Why this might happen
Unexplained	30%	This doesn't mean there *wasn't* a reason—our workup just wasn't able to identify it. I am hopeful that, with more awareness of the need for offering thorough investigations (as I describe below) as well as ongoing research that improves our understanding of stillbirth, this percentage will get closer to zero.
Infection	10–20%	Infections such as cytomegalovirus, parvovirus, Zika, Listeria, syphilis, and more.
Umbilical cord issues	10%	This can be hard to diagnose because about 25% of all babies are born with a cord around their neck (nuchal cord) and are fine. Sometimes in stillbirths, though, we can see very abnormal umbilical cords or ones with multiple loops around the neck, abnormal appearance, or tight knots that lead us to say this was the cause.
Birth defects or genetic disorders in the baby	5–15%	The most common is trisomy 21 (Down syndrome), but others can also lead to a loss.
Placental abruption	5–10%	Trauma (like a bad car accident), cocaine use, smoking, and preeclampsia can cause this.
Other (such as very severe growth restriction)		Multiple issues can contribute to problems like abnormal fetal growth, which can contribute to stillbirth, such as impaired placental development and function, genetic problems, high blood pressure, IVF pregnancies, smoking, and more.

In order to figure out what caused a loss, we usually discuss doing the following. **You need to know that your wishes are important and you aren't obligated to consent to all of these tests or procedures, but keep in mind some of these are time-dependent—so unfortunately it means needing to think about them before you leave the hospital.** Some people want every test done to try to figure out what happened, while others find that traumatizing. You decide what is best for you.

These are potential tests and procedures your medical team can do to help understand your baby's stillbirth better:

1. **Do an external exam of your baby.** Noting any developmental abnormalities that may have contributed. This can include taking pictures to keep in your baby's chart for future reference if needed.
2. **Examine the placenta.** Looking at it and the cord to see any abnormalities, and also sending it to the pathology lab to run tests for infection and look at it under a microscope for any signs of infection, blood vessel blockages, or other factors.
3. **Do genetic testing on your baby.** This can be done on your baby, placenta, and/or amniotic fluid. You can select all or some of these tests, which can include sending the following to a genetics lab:
    - A part of the umbilical cord
    - A part of the placenta
    - A tissue sample from your baby (this requires an incision often on the ankle, thigh, or elsewhere, but can be concealed with clothing afterward)
    - Amniotic fluid collected before delivery via an amniocentesis
4. **Do an internal exam of your baby,** which can include:
    - Autopsy
    - Imaging (i.e., X-ray, MRI, ultrasound)
5. **Take a detailed history from you.** The goal is to identify anything that could highlight genetic conditions, exposures to medications,

previous infections, or medical diagnoses that could play a role. This also may involve a referral to a genetic counselor.

6. **Do testing on you and your partner as indicated.** Depending on what the clinical situation is, your team may recommend:

    - Blood tests looking for signs that the baby bled into your bloodstream
    - Blood tests for infection
    - Blood tests for clotting disorders
    - Genetic testing for you and possibly your partner

It can be hard to make these decisions right after delivering your baby. What I've seen work well for my patients experiencing this is to talk about all these options even before we begin the labor process, so that we have time to talk for as long as we need. It also lets us get this out of the way so as not to interrupt your time after your baby is born.

I want you to know you can change your mind about any or all of these tests, and it's OK to ask as many questions as you need when you're trying to decide. You can also ask to have the options provided to you in writing to give you some time to review it with your loved ones.

WHAT CAN I DO TO COMMEMORATE MY BABY?

There are many things we can do to preserve the memory of your baby, and I bet there are even more that I haven't listed here. Here are some suggestions:

1. **Name your baby.** Naming your baby, and telling us so we can call them by their name, is one way to honor your baby. I have seen parents worry about using the name they wanted for a baby who is stillborn because they may want to "save" that name for a future

living child. It is perfectly OK to pivot and choose a new name—you are not a bad parent for having this thought.

2. **Footprints and handprints.** Once your baby is born, we can make commemorative prints. I have seen these made into beautiful tattoos and artwork. If possible, you may want to have a mold made of your baby's hands and feet too.

3. **Newborn photos.** Many hospitals partner with photographers who will come in any time, day or night, to take the most beautiful photos of your baby and give you something to remember them by. Now I Lay Me Down to Sleep is the main group, but local photographers or even some labor and delivery nurses who are talented at capturing these photos can do this. While these photos or videos may be hard to look at in the days immediately after your loss, you may want to consider capturing them so you can view them later when you feel emotionally ready. Many parents treasure them and often wish they had more.

4. **Bond with your baby.** Though your baby was born still, you can still care for them by bathing them, combing their hair, changing them into an outfit from home, and singing them lullabies. You can offer time for older siblings to talk to and have one-on-one time with the baby. You may want to wrap them in a blanket that you then bring home so you can keep something they've touched.

5. **Mementos.** We can give you a memory box filled with mementos of your baby that can include prints, their hat and baby blanket, and locks of hair. If you aren't planning on doing testing on the placenta, you can take it home and plant it under a tree or bush that commemorates your baby.

6. **Preserving their ashes.** If you choose to have your baby cremated, you can incorporate some of their ashes into jewelry and other keepsakes that can be deeply meaningful.

HOW DO I TELL MY OTHER CHILDREN?

This can feel like an insurmountable task, and I am sorry you have to do this. How you do it will depend on the age and temperament of your children, and what feels right for your family. These are some tips:

1. **Be honest and clear.** Younger kids especially are very concrete and won't understand nuanced terms. Using words like "died" instead of "born sleeping" or "went away" will help them know what happened. This can also prevent the stillbirth from being the basis of fears like being afraid to go to sleep at night.

2. **Let them see your emotions.** You do not need to "be strong" for your children; in fact, letting them see you cry or be angry gives them permission to have and share these feelings too.

3. **Make sure they know this isn't their fault.** Enough said on that.

4. **Allow them to be involved.** Offer to let them see and hold their baby brother or sister if this is possible, but do *not* pressure them. Honoring how much or little they want to be involved is important so as not to make them feel forced or guilty. Even the youngest kids should have this option, as it can help them understand what has happened.

5. **Give them chances to talk.** Whether it's immediately or even years later, giving them space to share how they feel is important and healthy. You can involve other friends, family members, or a child psychologist if you're hurting too much to listen at any time.

6. **Involve them in remembering your baby.** Whether it's a blessing before you leave the hospital, a reading at a funeral, hanging a stocking at Christmas, or remembering their birthday, involving

siblings can be a very healthy way to keep your baby's memory and their connection alive.

7. **Make sure others in your children's lives know what happened.** This includes their teachers, coaches, neighbors, and others. This is something you can task a friend or family member to communicate, if they ask for a way to help.
8. **Use the hospital resources.** Most hospitals will have a social worker or child life advocate who can come and help you tell your other children what happened. They are often very experienced at this and can help facilitate these conversations. They will often bring resources like children's books that talk about stillbirth to help both now and when you go home.

HOW AM I SUPPOSED TO LEAVE THE HOSPITAL WITHOUT MY BABY?

I can't pretend I know what this is like personally, but I can only imagine that this might be one of the darkest moments after having experienced a loss. To have to leave the hospital without a baby but rather a box of mementos, and to return home to where you have a nursery to face, must be an excruciating heartbreak.

I can only offer my support in the form of letting you know that you are not alone. Your grief is real, but how it affects you will change over time. I had this explained to me as the idea of grief being a rock in a jar. The size of the rock doesn't ever shrink, but the jar around it grows over time. That symbolizes that while your grief will never go away, you will have more capacity to feel joy in the future (represented by the size of the jar being bigger eventually).

Attempting to plan ahead for your return home may help. This could look like having someone help put away baby items before you go back, asking your best friend to be waiting for you in your house or to set up a meal train (you will be postpartum and, though grieving, you need nourishing meals), or asking family members to pitch in with childcare if you have other children, as you may not be ready to jump back into your daily routine right away. Or it could mean telling your network that you need time to yourself and you'll reach out when ready.

It can also be immensely helpful to involve the support of a therapist who specializes in perinatal loss, and other parents who have walked this path before. I share some suggestions at the end of this section that can help you connect to these resources.

WHERE DO I GO FROM HERE?

There's no one perfect answer for this, as everyone's situation and grief are unique. But in addition to physically healing from a vaginal birth or surgical procedure, you are also having to heal from the loss of your baby. You need and deserve so much extra support, and I don't want to shortchange you.

I want to highlight just a few things to be mindful of, but really I want you to get input from organizations and people who know exactly what you are experiencing. I'll list those resources here as well as at the end of this book so you can get the help and support you need.

1. **What to do with your milk.** After 20 weeks of pregnancy, your body will likely make some milk, and you may notice engorgement in the days after your pregnancy ends. This can be distressing if you don't expect it. You've got a few options when it comes to how to manage this:

- **Try to decrease your milk supply.** You can head to page 246, "I don't want to breastfeed, so what should I do?," for tips on getting more physical comfort.
- **Donate your breastmilk.** Whether it's a few drops or months' worth of pumping, milk banks can take your milk to help other vulnerable babies. This can be extremely healing for some parents who've lost their babies. I've got info in the resource list on the next page on how to see where you might be able to donate your milk.
- **Make keepsake breastmilk jewelry or mementos.** There are many companies that will take a small sample of your breastmilk (or ashes or a lock of hair) to make high-quality jewelry or pieces that you can keep to commemorate your baby.

2. **Please keep your postpartum visits.** I know it may seem impossible to go back to your OB-GYN and see all those pregnant bellies in the waiting room. A visit after a loss can be important, though, in us talking through what happened, any information we've gotten from our workup, what we might do in future pregnancies (if planned), and in making sure you are getting the support you need. You can definitely request a telehealth visit, or to be seen at the beginning or end of the day so that you needn't sit in the waiting room.

3. **Let us know if you are having thoughts of harming yourself.** You and your partner are at an increased risk for postpartum mood disorders (more on page 270). If you are having thoughts of hurting yourself, please let us know immediately, go to the nearest emergency department, call 911, or call the Suicide and Crisis Lifeline at 988. We are here to help, and this world is so much better with you in it.

Resource List

Below are some resources to get you started, but it is far from complete. For additional and updated resources, I recommend PUSH Pregnancy's website, which is frequently updated.

PUSH Pregnancy (their resource page is frequently updated and a great place to start): **https://www.pushpregnancy.org/loss**

March of Dimes: **https://www.marchofdimes.org/find-support/topics/miscarriage-loss-grief/stillbirth**

Aaliyah in Action (self-care boxes for moms): **https://www.aaliyahinaction.org**

Postpartum Support International (peer mentoring and virtual support groups): **https://www.postpartum.net/get-help/loss-grief-in-pregnancy-postpartum**

Managing milk after a loss: **https://www.pushpregnancy.org/post/lactation-after-stillbirth-tips-and-support**

Video for breast massage and hand expression after a loss: **https://vimeo.com/374979707**

Newborn photos: **https://www.nowilaymedowntosleep.org**

Star Legacy Foundation (organization focusing on stillbirth research, education, and support): **https://starlegacyfoundation.org/for-families-and-friends**

CONCLUSION

It's a lot, isn't it?

This is why I felt an entire book needed to be dedicated to "just" the part about having your baby—without even touching the pregnancy content! I wrote 293 pages and I am sure there's even more I could have covered.

I hope that this book has given you not only education but also a sense of control, a deeper understanding, and a true context of the labor and delivery you may experience. I hope it pulled back the curtain on what happens when you have a baby and lets you be prepared in a way that centers you and your human dignity in this life-changing process.

In short, I hope it empowers you to know what you can have and what you deserve as a pregnant person in this country.

I hope what you learned here helps you start conversations with your doctors, midwives, and nurses. Birth is a team sport—it isn't about telling someone what they have to do or assuming the person caring for you has ill intentions. We're all on the same side—or should be. If you feel otherwise, it's OK to seek out a new team.

But a word on teams: Great teams are built on honesty and assuming good intent. So, if you're worried because you're being told you need a blood transfusion or forceps or to transfer to a hospital and you have doubts, say that. Use this book to guide you. And if the doctor or midwife meets you in a place of honesty and transparency, know that sometimes plans digress without any agenda on anyone's part.

In my perfect world, you've read this book during your pregnancy.

You marked a couple of sections that stood out to you as important, and you used these to form your questions during your prenatal appointments. When the time comes to have your baby, you walk into Labor and Delivery nervous but excited, a little scared but prepared, and with the language to know what's happening and what to expect.

To doctors, nurses, or midwives reading this book: If you've found some of what I've written feels too out there or controversial, I get it. I also have come from a place of "this is how I was trained" or focusing on the risks that were unacceptable to me. Then I did this doctoring thing for a while... and realized I was missing some important perspectives: We haven't always gotten it right, and it's not always about us. I invite you to dive into the references I've provided. Chat with your colleagues. Think about the history of birthing in America and where some of our practices came from. Most importantly, think about our current outcomes and whether or not it seems to be working well. If the answer is no, then isn't it time we do something different?

Thank you so much for spending your precious time reading this book and allowing me to be a part of this journey you're on. Every birth is a story, and I wish you all the best in writing yours.

RESOURCES

You can access these resources and printable versions of checklists here: **https://www.drjenniferlincoln.com/books**

THE WHO AND THE WHERE

- State licensure of a doctor or midwife: **https://www.fsmb.org/contact-a-state-medical-board**
- Find a birth center: **https://www.birthcenters.org**
- Verify your CNM's or CM's credentials at the American Midwifery Certification Board: **https://www.amcbmidwife.org**
- For CPMs, you can make an inquiry at the North American Registry of Midwives: email support@narm.org
- Sample waterbirth consent and clinical policy: **https://onlinelibrary.wiley.com/doi/abs/10.1111/jmwh.12193**
- Find a doctor as a woman of color at Health in Her Hue: **https://healthinherhue.com**
- Find a certified doula at DONA International: **https://www.dona.org/what-is-a-doula-2/find-a-doula**
- VBAC calculator: **https://mfmunetwork.bsc.gwu.edu/web/mfmunetwork/vaginal-birth-after-cesarean-calculator**

WELCOME TO THE (BIRTHDAY) PARTY

- Sample protocol/statement on intermittent auscultation in labor: **https://ilpqc.org/ILPQC%202020+/PVB/Toolkit/FI/AWHONN%20Position%20Statement%20FH.pdf**

- Reference if you need a starting point to discuss eating in labor: **https://pmc.ncbi.nlm.nih.gov/articles/PMC7104541**

IF THINGS GET INTERESTING

- Preeclampsia Foundation: **https://www.preeclampsia.org**
- Information for you if you've had preeclampsia: **https://www.preeclampsia.org/beyondpregnancy**
- My Health Beyond Pregnancy handout for you and your primary care doctor if you've had preeclampsia: **https://www.preeclampsia.org/public/frontend/assets/img/gallery/pdf/My_Health_Beyond_Pregnancy_FINAL_2024.pdf**
- Postpartum preeclampsia information: **https://www.preeclampsia.org/postpartum-preeclampsia**

THE GRAND ENTRANCE (OR EXIT)

- Position changes for moving an OP baby: **https://www.spinningbabies.com/pregnancy-birth/baby-position/posterior**
- Check your hospital's episiotomy rates: **https://ratings.leapfroggroup.org**
- Find a public bank to donate cord blood to: **https://www.nmdp.org/what-we-do/partnerships/global-transplant-network/cord-blood-banks-and-hospitals**
- Vaccine information: **https://www.chop.edu/vaccine-update-healthcare-professionals/resources/vaccine-and-vaccine-safety-related-qa-sheets**

THE AFTERPARTY

- Breastfeeding resources:
    - This directory can help you find an IBCLC in your community: **https://portal.ilca.org/i4a/memberDirectory/index.cfm?directory_id=19&pageID=4356**

- La Leche League USA: **https://lllusa.org**
- KellyMom (parenting and breastfeeding support): **https://kellymom.com**
- Stanford Medicine Newborn Nursery (getting started with breastfeeding with fantastic videos on hand expression, well-fed baby checklist, and more): **https://med.stanford.edu/newborns/professional-education/breastfeeding.html**
- National Women's Health and Breastfeeding Helpline: free help with breastfeeding or other health issues (in English and Spanish) 9 A.M. to 6 P.M. EST, Monday through Friday, at 1-800-994-9662
- **https://womenshealth.gov/about-us/what-we-do/programs-and-activities/helpline**
- InfantRisk Center: free call center staffed with experts about questions regarding medications and breastfeeding, Monday through Friday, 8 A.M. to 3 P.M. CST at 1-806-352-2519; also **https://www.infantrisk.com/infantrisk-center-resources**
- MommyMeds app (from the Texas Tech University Health Sciences Center's InfantRisk Center, this app has up-to-date information about prescription and over-the-counter medications and their safety during pregnancy and breastfeeding): **https://apps.apple.com/us/app/mommymeds/id669222544**
- Breastmilk storage tips from the CDC: **https://www.cdc.gov/breastfeeding/breast-milk-preparation-and-storage/handling-breastmilk.html**
- WIC Going Back to Work tips: **https://wicbreastfeeding.fns.usda.gov/going-back-to-work**

- Bedsider (birth control information): **https://www.bedsider.org**
- Postpartum emergency warning signs printable poster: **https://pbws.s3.amazonaws.com/PBWSSaveYourLifeHandout_English.pdf**

- Postpartum mental health resources:
    - Suicide and Crisis Lifeline: call 988 (24 hours a day, 7 days a week, 365 days a year) or go to **https://988lifeline.org**
    - Postpartum Support International: **www.postpartum.net**
- Birth trauma resources:
    - Make Birth Better (UK-based group with excellent informational PDFs): **https://www.makebirthbetter.org**
    - Postpartum Support International (resources and free online support groups, including a BIPOC birth trauma group): **https://postpartum.net**
    - Birth Trauma Association (UK-based group with amazing amounts of information): **https://www.birthtraumaassociation.org**

STILLBIRTH

- PUSH Pregnancy (their resource page is frequently updated and a great place to start): **https://www.pushpregnancy.org/loss**
- March of Dimes: **https://www.marchofdimes.org/find-support/topics/miscarriage-loss-grief/stillbirth**
- Aaliyah in Action (self-care boxes for moms): **https://www.aaliyahinaction.org**
- Postpartum Support International (peer mentoring and virtual support groups): **https://www.postpartum.net/get-help/loss-grief-in-pregnancy-postpartum**
- Managing milk after a loss: **https://www.pushpregnancy.org/post/lactation-after-stillbirth-tips-and-support**
- Video showing breast massage and hand expression after a loss: **https://vimeo.com/374979707**
- Newborn photos: **https://www.nowilaymedowntosleep.org**
- Star Legacy Foundation (organization focusing on stillbirth research, education, and support): **https://starlegacyfoundation.org/for-families-and-friends**

BIRTH PREFERENCES

Name:

Doctor/midwife:

Primary support person/relationship:

Doula:

Additional support people:

The three things that are most important for you to know about myself and the arrival of baby (name) ______________________________ are:

1.

2.

3.

Please discuss the following with me when I get admitted so I can ask questions before an urgent situation arises:

[ ] Operative vaginal delivery (vacuum and forceps)

[ ] C-section

[ ] Blood transfusion

[ ] ____

Pain management:

[ ] Please explain all my medication options

[ ] Please do not offer any medications unless I ask

[ ] I would like non-drug options offered (birthing ball, tub/shower, etc.)

[ ] I am planning an epidural

[ ] I would like to meet the anesthesia team to discuss my epidural on admission, so I am not in pain when I go through the consent process

[ ] ______________________________

Labor preferences:

[ ] I would like to be free to move around in labor in positions that feel best for me

I would like to be offered

[ ] birthing ball
[ ] whirlpool bath/tub
[ ] birthing stool for laboring

[ ] I prefer intermittent fetal monitoring if it is not too risky for me

[ ] I prefer wireless monitoring if it is available

[ ] I want to be able to eat and drink

[ ] I do not want routine breaking of the bag of water or internal monitoring; if they are recommended, I want the reasoning explained to me

[ ] I do not want routine Pitocin during labor; if it is recommended, I want the reason explained to me

[ ] I decline scheduled cervical exams and instead want them when there is a clinical reason and it is explained to me first

[ ] ______________________________

Pushing preferences:

[ ] I would like to push and birth my baby in whatever position feels right and is safe and effective (this may not be on my back!)

[ ] I want warm compresses on my perineum when I'm pushing

I want perineal massage

- [ ] while pushing
- [ ] in between pushes
- [ ] both

[ ] I would like a mirror when I am pushing

I prefer pushing to be

- [ ] coached
- [ ] uncoached
- [ ] whatever you think is working best

[ ] If my baby appears to be sunny side up while pushing, I would like to discuss the potential benefits of trying manual rotation

[ ] ______________________________

Birthing preferences:

[ ] I want my baby placed skin-to-skin right after birth, and for them to remain there during the golden hour (unless their or my medical condition prevents that)

[ ] If I am unable to do skin-to-skin for the first hour, I would like ______________________________ to do this

[ ] I decline routine bulb suctioning and only want it done if my baby's airway needs to be cleared

[ ] ______________________________

Umbilical cord and placenta preferences:

[ ] I would like delayed cord clamping of at least sixty seconds

[ ] I would like to donate the cord blood to public banking if it is available

[ ] I do not want to take my placenta home with me

[ ] I want to take my placenta home with me

[ ] I would like to be shown my placenta

[ ] I plan to have a post-placental IUD placed

[ ] ______________________________

C-section preferences:

[ ] If a C-section is recommended, I would like the reason explained to me and the ability to ask if we can try alternatives (understanding that emergencies sometimes happen and limit this)

I want a clear drape

- [ ] so I can watch my baby be born
- [ ] only after my baby is out, to see them
- [ ] I do not want to see anything until after my baby is born and brought over to me

[ ] I want delayed cord clamping

[ ] I want the umbilical cord left long so __________ can cut it afterward

[ ] I want my baby immediately brought to me and assessed while on my chest during skin-to-skin, unless a medical concern prevents this

[ ] I do not want my baby to leave the operating room unless it is medically necessary

I prefer my skin incision be closed with

- [ ] stitches
- [ ] staples
- [ ] whatever my doctor recommends

Baby preferences:

[ ] I want all procedures (including shots/eye ointment) to wait until after the golden hour has passed

[ ] I want my baby to be given all routine vaccinations and medications

I do not want my baby given a bath

- [ ] until 24 hours old
- [ ] while in the hospital
- [ ] I want my baby rooming in with me and all examinations and testing done in my presence

[ ] If I have a boy, I would like to discuss circumcision

Feeding preferences:

I plan to

- [ ] exclusively breastfeed
- [ ] combination feed
- [ ] exclusively formula-feed

[ ] I do not want any supplementation given without my consent

If supplementation is needed, I prefer

- [ ] donor breastmilk
- [ ] formula
- [ ] want to see the hospital lactation consultant

CHECKLISTS

WHAT TO ASK YOUR DOCTOR/MIDWIFE PRENATALLY

1. Do you take my insurance?
2. What hospital(s) do you deliver babies at?
3. How do I get in touch with you after hours/on weekends?
4. Is there an online portal for questions/results/scheduling?
5. Are there males in the practice (*if this matters to you*)?
6. Will I see medical students, midwifery students, residents, or other learners?
7. Do you partner with midwives?
8. Are you OK with me having a doula?
9. Who can I expect to see in the hospital and at my birth?
10. Is there an OB hospitalist present 24/7 on Labor and Delivery?
11. Can I take photos? Video?
12. What is your C-section rate? Episiotomy rate?
13. If I need a C-section:
    - Can my support person be in the operating room with me? Will you use a clear drape so I can see my baby once they're born?
    - Can you confirm my baby won't leave the operating room unless there is an issue?
    - Will you close my incision with stitches or staples?

14. Am I able to have a trial of labor after cesarean (TOLAC) if I want that?

15. Do you use forceps or vacuum, or both? What is your rate of using these?

16. If my baby is breech, is an external cephalic version and/or vaginal breech birth something you offer?

17. What's your philosophy on cervical exams and how often they're done?

18. How do you feel about birth plans/preferences?

19. If I want to do the following, are you supportive of:

    - Intermittent monitoring if I am low-risk?
    - Laboring, pushing, or birthing in positions that feel best for me, including being upright or off my back?

20. Is delayed cord clamping and immediate skin-to-skin standard in your practice and that of your partners?

21. If I want my tubes tied or have an IUD or arm implant birth control placed after I give birth, would you be able to do that?

WHAT TO ASK ABOUT YOUR HOSPITAL

1. Does my insurance cover this hospital? And everyone who works in it?

2. Can you care for my baby if they are born preterm? Or is there a gestational age cutoff below which you'd have to transfer my baby to a different hospital?

3. Is an anesthesiologist and operating room team available and physically present in the hospital 24/7?

4. Is the anesthesiologist employed by the hospital? Do they take my insurance? Or is it a separate contracted group?
5. What is the C-section rate for the hospital?
6. Do you offer doulas? If not, am I able to have my own doula present?
7. Does the hospital have a blood bank that carries all blood products, or only some?
8. Am I able to donate my baby's cord blood to a public bank?
9. If I want to take home my placenta, is that going to be an issue?
10. What are my options for pain relief besides an epidural, such as nitrous oxide?
11. Are midwives present on Labor and Delivery, and how do they work with the physicians?
12. Does the hospital offer tours and/or birth and breastfeeding prep classes?
13. Can my pediatrician see my baby in the hospital, or does a hospital-employed pediatrician care for all babies?
14. Do you offer tubs or whirlpool baths for laboring in? How likely is it that one will be available for me to use?
15. Is waterbirth an option?
16. Is wireless fetal monitoring an option?
17. Is an OB hospitalist present on the unit 24/7?
18. If I have a C-section, am I able to do skin-to-skin in the OR?
19. What is the visitor policy?
20. Is this a designated baby-friendly hospital?

21. What breastfeeding help is available to me?

22. Do babies room in, and if so, is there a respite nursery if I need a break?

23. What is the hospital's policy on the timing of newborn baths?

24. Is there access to donor milk if I need to supplement, and if so, is it available for anyone or reserved for certain babies like those in the NICU?

25. Am I able to get comprehensive reproductive care, such as an abortion if needed or a tubal ligation after I have my baby, or are there religious restrictions?

WHAT TO ASK YOUR HOMEBIRTH/ BIRTH CENTER MIDWIFE

1. What's the hospital you recommend if I need to be transferred in labor? How close is it? What kind of relationship do you have with the medical team there? How have your patients felt treated by them? Will they allow you to come with me and stay as a support person?

2. What supplies and resources do you have here if we need them (i.e., medications for pain or bleeding, resuscitative equipment for baby)?

3. How many births have you attended? What is your licensing? Do you have references for patients I can contact to discuss their experience here? Can I see your statistics on transfers and complications?

4. Who is here to help you during my labor and birth? And who covers you if you're with another patient? Where do I go if the center here is full?

5. Are you able to give me antibiotics if I have group B strep? Rho-gam if needed? Baby medications like vitamin K, eye ointment, and newborn vaccines?

6. What criteria do you use to make sure I am safe to birth here?

Additionally, check the following:

- Check with your state's medical board to see what is allowed in your state (i.e., can midwives prescribe or carry lifesaving medications, etc.).
- Verify your midwife's credentials at the American Midwifery Certification Board.

WHAT TO ASK YOUR PEDIATRICIAN

1. How accessible are you and how easy is it to make appointments?

    a. Can I schedule an appointment for an acute issue on the same day?
    b. Is the clinic open on weekends?
    c. Who answers the phone during business hours when I have a clinical question? What happens if I have a question in the middle of the night?
    d. Do you have an online portal where I can send in questions?
    e. Do you offer telehealth visits?
    f. How many days a week do you see patients?
    g. If I'm not seeing you, who fills in?

2. Will I see you in the hospital when my baby is born?

3. What support can I expect at your clinic?

    a. Do you have a lactation consultant, a social worker, therapists, or behavioral specialists available?

   b. If I need referrals elsewhere, do you have someone who coordinates this and makes it easy?

4. What is your communication style?
5. What's the best part of your job?
6. Can you help with my medically complex child?
   a. Have you taken care of kids with ___ issue before? *(if you have a concern with certain issues or a prenatal diagnosis you know about)*
   b. Do you know the pediatric subspecialists and can you help with referrals and care coordination?

WHAT TO PACK CHECKLIST

What you should bring
Your ID
Your insurance card
Baby car seat (before discharge)
A copy of your birth plan/preferences
This book!
What can be nice to have
Stuff to keep you entertained (especially during a labor induction!): a book, magazine, your laptop, etc., and all chargers
Stuff to keep you comfy: a playlist, some battery-powered candles, personal toiletries, slippers, bathrobe or PJs you don't mind throwing out after, a white noise machine/ phone app (the hospital can be noisy)
Stuff to keep you full: snacks or drinks that you like
Stuff for after: a comfy nursing bra, an outfit for your baby, and a maternity outfit for you going home (regular clothes won't fit yet—that's OK!)

ACKNOWLEDGMENTS

With any pregnancy and birth, it takes a team to get the best outcome—and the same can be said for writing a book.

First and foremost, I want to thank my agent, Joy Tutela of the David Black Literary Agency, who one day seemingly out of the blue sent me an email asking if I was ready to start writing my next book. It was as if she'd read my mind and knew I'd been thinking about it just that week, and her question was the final nudge I needed to start working on *The Birth Book*. Thank you for always being in my corner and supporting me throughout this process.

I also want to thank my editor, Michele Eniclerico, whose feedback and assistance was always spot-on. I also need to thank Marnie Cochran, who filled in for Michele's editorial duties while Michele was out on maternity leave (and yes, I love that my editor was the exact target audience for this book and even more reason I'm so glad she was alongside me in this process!). To the entire Rodale team, from copyediting to proofreading to design to PR and marketing: Thank you so much for helping me bring this work to life.

To Liz Paton, my illustrator, who immediately saw my vision when I described what I wanted: Thank you for your work. You are so talented, and so many pregnant patients are going to have their babies with a clearer understanding because of the images you created. I hope we get to connect in Glasgow one day!

To Ashley Sandberg and the entire Triple 7 PR team: Thank you for being so amazing at what you do and helping more pregnant folks know this resource exists. I'm so glad we finally got to work together.

I am indebted to the many expert reviewers who took the time to review sections of this book and provide detailed, thoughtful feedback. Their input was invaluable, and any errors are mine alone. Thank you to licensed direct entry midwife and certified professional midwife Emilia Smith, OB hospitalist and Society of OB/GYN Hospitalists past president (and featured simulation actress in this book) Dr. Vanessa Torbenson, doula extraordinaire Rauna Otteson, labor and delivery nurse and social media educator Liesel Teen (aka **@mommy.labornurse**), OB hospitalist and wonderful colleague Dr. Hallie Stosur, maternal-fetal medicine specialist and friend Dr. Laura Sienas, rockstar certified nurse midwife Ashlee Walter, registered nurse and president of the Association of Women's Health, Obstetric and Neonatal Nurses Rose Horton, OB-GYN/stellar human/past president of the American College of Obstetricians and Gynecologists Dr. Stella Dantas, labor and delivery nurse and night shift partner in crime Suni Hughes, OB hospitalist Dr. Kathy Jorda, International Board Certified Lactation Consultant Melissa Cole, urogynecologist/advocate for our specialty Dr. Jocelyn Fitzgerald, anesthesiologist Dr. Melissa Duan (I miss working with you!), OB hospitalist and remarkable advocate for community/hospital birth collaboration Dr. Wendy Davis, and Ana Lepe Vick, director of communications at PUSH for Empowered Pregnancy and mom to Owen Nathaniel Vick, who was born still on October 3, 2015.

To my wonderful community on social media, thank you for engaging with my content and letting me know what I need to cover. The internet can be an interesting place, but I have definitely seen the positive side of it and am thankful for all of you who follow along.

I also must thank my little sister Emily Hartman (Zeta is forever!), who, while on our trip to Germany that coincided with me selling my book, never once complained about having to entertain herself around Munich while I took over the hotel room with publisher meetings. I should also mention that while in Munich, we saw Taylor Swift on the Eras Tour, so perhaps I should also thank her for being the reward for the hard work—and if you ever have a baby, please read my book and let's be friends?

I wrote this book in the early mornings, stolen free moments during the day, on airplanes, and in coffee shops across Portland, but my favorite spot was the Reed College library. Thank you for opening your space to the community, and if any Reedies ever need this book, just be sure to let me know . . .

Thank you to my parents, who always made me feel I could do whatever I put my mind to. I am the advocate I am today because you always taught me to work hard and speak up for what is right.

To my boys, who asked such sweet questions about what writing a book is like and who understand some of the complex topics we talk about better than some adults I know: Thank you for understanding when Mom is on a meeting, or Mom is writing, or Mom is post-call and needs to sleep. Writing this book frequently brought me back to two of the best days of my life, which were when you both entered the world.

To my husband, Doug, who not only supported me throughout this whole process but also contributed to key sections with his expert pediatrician input: Your patients are so lucky to have such a smart, kind doctor who cares about them. I promise not to ask you any more questions about hepatitis B.

Thank you to my colleagues, who are the best OB hospitalists a girl could hope to work with. I am so thankful to be part of a group of physicians who always practice the compassionate, evidence-based care that I describe as the goal in this book. And endless thanks to all the folks on my unit—the nurses, midwives, surgical techs, doulas, anesthesiologists, lactation consultants, NICU team, social workers, and more. You are stellar people who come to work every day ready to care for and deal with whatever comes your way. Our country would be in a much better place if everyone received the quality of care that our team provides, and I hope this book can be a part of communicating what our patients want and deserve.

Lastly, but certainly not least, to the patients I have cared for and will get to care for in the future: Thank you for allowing me to be part of your birth story. I know many times we have met in emergency situations or right at the very end of your pregnancy, but I hope the care you received made you feel safe, seen, and heard. I learn so much from each of you and am indebted to the trust you place in me. I hope this book is a step toward making birth better in this country. Know that I will keep fighting for you every day of my career.

REFERENCES

Introduction

1. Stoneburner A, Lucas R, Fontenot J, Brigance C, Jones E, DeMaria AL. Nowhere to go: maternity care deserts across the US. Report no. 4. March of Dimes. 2024. **https://www.marchofdimes.org/maternity-care-deserts-report**

The Who and the Where

WHERE CAN I HAVE MY BABY?

1. American Association of Birth Centers. National BC Study II. 2013 Jan 31. **https://www.birthcenters.org/news/nbcs2**
2. American College of Obstetricians and Gynecologists. Planned home birth (committee opinion). 2017 Apr; reaffirmed 2023. **https://www.acog.org/clinical/clinical-guidance/committee-opinion/articles/2017/04/planned-home-birth**
3. Cheyney M, Bovbjerg ML, Leeman L, Vedam S. Community versus out-of-hospital birth: what's in a name? J Midwifery Womens Health. 2019 Jan;64(1):9–11. doi: 10.1111/jmwh.12947
4. Johnson KC, Daviss B. Outcomes of planned home births with certified professional midwives: large prospective study in North America. BMJ. 2005 Jun 18;330(7505):1416. doi: 10.1136/bmj.330.7505.1416
5. American Association of Birth Centers website. **https://www.birthcenters.org**

WHO CAN HELP ME DELIVER MY BABY?

1. American College of Obstetricians and Gynecologists. Midwifery education and certification (statement of policy). 2020 Nov; reaffirmed 2023 Jul. **https://www.acog.org/clinical-information/policy-and-position-statements/statements-of-policy/2020/midwifery-education-and-certification**
2. American Midwifery Certification Board website. **https://www.amcbmidwife.org/home**
3. American College of Nurse-Midwives. Comparison of Certified Nurse

Midwives, Certified Midwives, and Certified Professional Midwives. **https://www.midwife.org/acnm/files/cclibraryfiles/filename/000000008490/20220418_CNM-CM-CPM%20Comparison%20Chart_FINAL.pdf**

4. Oregon Affiliate of the American College of Nurse-Midwives. ACNM is the professional organization that represents Certified Nurse-Midwives (CNMs) and Certified Midwives (CMs) in the United States. **https://www.oregonmidwives.org/different-types-of-midwives**
5. North American Registry of Midwives. CPM eligibility review: focus group, survey, and outcomes. **https://narm.org/about/the-cpm-credential/eligibility-review**
6. American Association of Naturopathic Midwives website. **http://www.naturopathicmidwives.com**
7. Network for Public Health Law. Direct entry midwives across the nation. 2023 Apr. **https://www.networkforphl.org/wp-content/uploads/2023/05/Direct-Entry-Midwives-50-State-Survey.pdf**
8. Smith TM. What's the difference between physicians and naturopaths? American Medical Association. 2024 Feb 26. **https://www.ama-assn.org/practice-management/scope-practice/whats-difference-between-physicians-and-naturopaths**
9. American Association of Naturopathic Physicians. Regulated states and regulatory authorities. 2024 Jun. **https://naturopathic.org/page/RegulatedStates**

SHOULD I HAVE A WATERBIRTH?

1. American College of Obstetricians and Gynecologists. Approaches to limit intervention during labor and birth (committee opinion). 2019 Feb; reaffirmed 2021. **https://www.acog.org/clinical/clinical-guidance/committee-opinion/articles/2019/02/approaches-to-limit-intervention-during-labor-and-birth**
2. Nolt D, O'Leary ST, Aucott SW, Committee on Infectious Diseases and Committee on Fetus and Newborn. Risks of infectious diseases in newborns exposed to alternative perinatal practices. Pediatrics. 2022 Feb 1;149(2):e2021055554. doi: 10.1542/peds.2021-055554
3. McKinney JA, et al. Water birth: a systematic review and meta-analysis of maternal and neonatal outcomes. Am J Obstet Gynecol. 2024 Mar;230(3S):S961–S979.e33. doi: 10.1016/j.ajog.2023.08.034
4. Nutter E, Shaw-Battista J, Marowitz A. Waterbirth fundamentals for clinicians. J Midwifery Womens Health. 2014 May–Jun;59(3):350–4. doi: 10.1111/jmwh.12193
5. Peacock PJ, Zengeya ST, Cochrane L, Sleath M. Neonatal outcomes following delivery in water: evaluation of safety in a district general hospital. Cureus. 2018 Feb 20;10(2):e2208. doi: 10.7759/cureus.2208

WILL MY INSURANCE FOR MY OB-GYN COVER EVERYTHING . . . LIKE MY EPIDURAL?

1. Taylor EA, Parast L. A tale of two deliveries, or an out-of-network problem. Rand. 2015 Nov 4. **https://www.rand.org/pubs/commentary/2015/11/a-tale-of-two-deliveries-or-an-out-of-network-problem.html**

DOES THE RELIGIOUS AFFILIATION OF MY HOSPITAL MATTER?

1. US Conference of Catholic Bishops. Ethical and religious directives for Catholic health care services. 6th ed. 2018 Jun. **https://www.usccb.org/resources/ethical-religious-directives-catholic-health-service-sixth-edition-2016-06_0.pdf**
2. Pradhan R, Recht H. The powerful constraints on medical care in Catholic hospitals across America. Health News Florida. 2024 Feb 20. **https://health.wusf.usf.edu/health-news-florida/2024-02-20/the-powerful-constraints-on-medical-care-in-catholic-hospitals-across-america**
3. Takahashi J, Cher A, Sheeder J, Teal S, Guiahi M. Disclosure of religious identity and health care practices on Catholic hospital websites. JAMA. 2019 Mar 19;321(11):1103–1104. doi: 10.1001/jama.2019.0133

DOES THE RACE OF MY DOCTOR MATTER?

1. Blackstock U. Legacy: a black physician reckons with racism in medicine. 2024; Penguin. **https://books.google.com/books/about/Legacy.html?id=muqfEAAAQBAJ**
2. Salifu M, Clare CA, Minkoff H. Racism as a modifiable risk factor for adverse pregnancy outcomes. Am J Obstet Gynecol. 2024 Aug;231(2):150–151. doi: 10.1016/j.ajog.2024.02.292
3. Hill L, Rao A, Artiga S, Ranji U. Racial disparities in maternal and infant health: current status and efforts to address them. KFF. 2024 Oct 25. **https://www.kff.org/racial-equity-and-health-policy/issue-brief/racial-disparities-in-maternal-and-infant-health-current-status-and-efforts-to-address-them**
4. Greenwood BN, Hardeman RR, Huang L, Sojourner A. Physician-patient racial concordance and disparities in birthing mortality for newborns. Proc Natl Acad Sci USA. 117 (35) 21194–21200. **https://www.pnas.org/doi/10.1073/pnas.1913405117**
5. Preeclampsia Foundation. Preeclampsia and racial and ethnic disparities. 2020. **https://www.preeclampsia.org/public/frontend/assets/img/gallery/D0900705.pdf**

6. Association of American Medical Groups. U.S. physician workforce data dashboard. 2025. **https://www.aamc.org/data-reports/report/us-physician-workforce-data-dashboard.**
7. Association of American Medical Colleges. How we fail black patients in pain. 2020. **https://www.aamc.org/news/how-we-fail-black-patients-pain**
8. Kavattur PS, et al. The rise of pregnancy criminalization: a Pregnancy Justice report. 2023.

DO I NEED A DOULA?

1. DONA International. What is a doula? **https://www.dona.org/what-is-a-doula-2**
2. Bohren MA, Hofmeyr GJ, Sakala C, Fukuzawa RK, Cuthbert A. Continuous support for women during childbirth. Cochrane Database Syst Rev. 2017 Jul 6;7(7):CD003766. doi: 10.1002/14651858.CD003766.pub6. **https://www.ncbi.nlm.nih.gov/pmc/articles/PMC6483123**

CAN I JUST REQUEST A C-SECTION?

1. American College of Obstetricians and Gynecologists. Cesarean delivery on maternal request (committee opinion). 2019 Jan; reaffirmed 2024.
2. Barca JA, Bravo C, Pintado-Recarte MP, Asúnsolo Á, Cueto-Hernández I, Ruiz-Labarta J, Buján J, Ortega MA, De León-Luis JA. Pelvic floor morbidity following vaginal delivery versus cesarean delivery: systematic review and meta-analysis. J Clin Med. 2021 Apr 13;10(8):1652. doi: 10.3390/jcm10081652
3. Fitzpatrick KE, Abdel-Fattah M, Hemelaar J, Kurinczuk JJ, Quigley MA. Planned mode of birth after previous cesarean section and risk of undergoing pelvic floor surgery: a Scottish population-based record linkage cohort study. PLoS Med. 2022 Nov 22;19(11):e1004119. doi: 10.1371/journal.pmed.1004119
4. American College of Obstetricians and Gynecologists. Vaginal birth after cesarean delivery on maternal request (practice bulletin). 2019 Feb. **https://www.acog.org/clinical/clinical-guidance/practice-bulletin/articles/2019/02/vaginal-birth-after-cesarean-delivery**

IF I'VE HAD A C-SECTION BEFORE, SHOULD I HAVE ONE AGAIN?

1. American College of Obstetricians and Gynecologists. Vaginal birth after cesarean delivery on maternal request (practice bulletin). 2019 Feb. **https://www.acog.org/clinical/clinical-guidance/practice-bulletin/articles/2019/02/vaginal-birth-after-cesarean-delivery**

2. Guise JM, Denman MA, Emeis C, Marshall N, Walker M, Fu R, Janik R, Nygren P, Eden KB, McDonagh M. Vaginal birth after cesarean: new insights on maternal and neonatal outcomes. Obstet Gynecol. 2010 Jun;115(6):1267–1278. doi: 10.1097/AOG.0b013e3181df925f

Is It Time?

SHOULD I RUSH TO THE HOSPITAL IF MY BAG OF WATER BROKE BUT I'M NOT HAVING CONTRACTIONS?

1. American College of Obstetricians and Gynecologists. Prelabor rupture of membranes (practice bulletin). 2020 Mar. **https://www.acog.org/clinical/clinical-guidance/practice-bulletin/articles/2020/03/prelabor-rupture-of-membranes**
2. Middleton P, Shepherd E, Flenady V, McBain RD, Crowther CA. Planned early birth versus expectant management (waiting) for prelabour rupture of membranes at term (37 weeks or more). Cochrane Database Syst Rev. 2017 Jan 4;1(1):CD005302. doi: 10.1002/14651858.CD005302.pub3

WHAT DO I DO IF I GO PAST MY DUE DATE?

1. American College of Obstetricians and Gynecologists. Definition of term delivery (committee opinion). 2013 Nov. **https://www.acog.org/clinical/clinical-guidance/committee-opinion/articles/2013/11/definition-of-term-pregnancy**
2. American College of Obstetricians and Gynecologists. Management of late and post-term pregnancies (practice bulletin). 2014 Aug; reaffirmed 2024.
3. Muglu J, Rather H, Arroyo-Manzano D, Bhattacharya S, Balchin I, Khalil A, Thilaganathan B, Khan KS, Zamora J, Thangaratinam S. Risks of stillbirth and neonatal death with advancing gestation at term: a systematic review and meta-analysis of cohort studies of 15 million pregnancies. PLoS Med. 2019 Jul 2;16(7):e1002838. **https://journals.plos.org/plosmedicine/article?id=10.1371%2Fjournal.pmed.1002838**
4. Finucane EM, Murphy DJ, Biesty LM, Gyte GML, Cotter AM, Ryan EM, Boulvain M, Devane D. Membrane sweeping for induction of labour. Cochrane Database Syst Rev. 2020 Feb 27;2(2):CD000451. doi: 10.1002/14651858.CD000451.pub3
5. Smith CA. Homoeopathy for induction of labour. Cochrane Database Syst Rev. 2001;2003(4):CD003399. doi: 10.1002/14651858.CD003399
6. Kelly AJ, Kavanagh J, Thomas J. Castor oil, bath and/or enema for cervical priming and induction of labour. Cochrane Database Syst Rev. 2013 Jul 24;2013(7):CD003099. doi: 10.1002/14651858.CD003099.pub2

7. Smith CA, Collins CT, Levett KM, Armour M, Dahlen HG, Tan AL, Mesgarpour B. Acupuncture or acupressure for pain management during labour. Cochrane Database Syst Rev. 2020 Feb 7;2(2):CD009232. doi: 10.1002/14651858.CD009232.pub2
8. Kavanagh J, Kelly AJ, Thomas J. Sexual intercourse for cervical ripening and induction of labour. Cochrane Database Syst Rev. 2001;2001(2):CD003093. doi: 10.1002/14651858.CD003093
9. Muglu J, Rather H, Arroyo-Manzano D, Bhattacharya S, Balchin I, Khalil A, Thilaganathan B, Khan KS, Zamora J, Thangaratinam S. Risks of stillbirth and neonatal death with advancing gestation at term: a systematic review and meta-analysis of cohort studies of 15 million pregnancies. PLoS Med. 2019 Jul 2;16(7):e1002838. **https://doi.org/10.1371/journal.pmed.1002838**
10. Salajegheh Z, Nasiri M, Imanipour M, Zamanifard M, Sadeghi O, Ghasemi Dehcheshmeh M, Asadi M. Is oral consumption of dates (Phoenix dactylifera L. fruit) in the peripartum period effective and safe integrative care to facilitate childbirth and improve perinatal outcomes: a comprehensive revised systematic review and dose-response meta-analysis. BMC Pregnancy Childbirth. 2024 Jan 2;24(1):12. **https://doi.org/10.1186/s12884-023-06196-y**

Welcome to the (Birthday) Party

WHAT ARE THE REASONS I CAN GET ADMITTED TO LABOR AND DELIVERY?

1. American College of Obstetricians and Gynecologists. First and second stage labor management (clinical practice guideline). 2024 Jan. **https://www.acog.org/clinical/clinical-guidance/clinical-practice-guideline/articles/2024/01/first-and-second-stage-labor-management**

MY DOCTOR WANTS TO INDUCE MY LABOR. SHOULD I?

1. Simpson KR. Trends in labor induction in the United States, 1989 to 2020. MCN Am J Matern Child Nurs. 2022 Jul–Aug 01;47(4):235. doi: 10.1097/NMC.0000000000000824
2. American College of Obstetricians and Gynecologists. Induction of labor (practice bulletin). 2009 Aug. **https://www.acog.org/clinical/clinical-guidance/practice-bulletin/articles/2009/08/induction-of-labor**
3. American College of Obstetricians and Gynecologists. Management of late-term and postterm pregnancies (practice bulletin). 2014 Aug. **https://www.acog.org/clinical/clinical-guidance/practice-bulletin/articles/2014/08/management-of-late-term-and-postterm-pregnancies**

4. American College of Obstetricians and Gynecologists. Medically indicated late-preterm and early-term deliveries (committee opinion). 2021 Jul. **https://www.acog.org/clinical/clinical-guidance/committee-opinion/articles/2021/07/medically-indicated-late-preterm-and-early-term-deliveries**
5. American College of Obstetricians and Gynecologists. Macrosomia (practice bulletin). 2020 Jan. **https://www.acog.org/clinical/clinical-guidance/practice-bulletin/articles/2020/01/macrosomia**

MY DOCTOR SAYS A TRIAL SHOWED IT'S SAFEST TO GIVE BIRTH AT 39 WEEKS, SO SHOULD I BE INDUCED THEN?

1. Grobman WA, Rice MM, Reddy UM, Tita ATN, Silver RM, Mallett G, Hill K, Thom EA, El-Sayed YY, Perez-Delboy A, Rouse DJ, Saade GR, Boggess KA, Chauhan SP, Iams JD, Chien EK, Casey BM, Gibbs RS, Srinivas SK, Swamy GK, Simhan HN, Macones GA; Eunice Kennedy Shriver National Institute of Child Health and Human Development Maternal–Fetal Medicine Units Network. Labor induction versus expectant management in low-risk nulliparous women. N Engl J Med. 2018 Aug 9;379(6):513–523. **https://www.nejm.org/doi/full/10.1056/NEJMoa1800566**
2. SMFM statement on elective induction of labor in low-risk nulliparous women at term: the ARRIVE trial. Am J Obstet Gynecol. 2019 Jul;221(1): B2–B4
3. Management of full-term nulliparous individuals without a medical indication for delivery: ACOG clinical practice update. Obstet Gynecol. 2025 Jan 1;145(1):e45–e50. doi: 10.1097/AOG.0000000000005783

I'VE BEEN TOLD I NEED AN INDUCTION OF LABOR—HOW LONG DOES THIS TAKE?

1. American College of Obstetricians and Gynecologists. Induction of labor (practice bulletin). 2009 Aug. **https://www.acog.org/clinical/clinical-guidance/practice-bulletin/articles/2009/08/induction-of-labor**

HOW DOES AN INDUCTION WORK?

1. American College of Obstetricians and Gynecologists. Induction of labor (practice bulletin). 2009 Aug. **https://www.acog.org/clinical/clinical-guidance/practice-bulletin/articles/2009/08/induction-of-labor**
2. Kavanagh J, Kelly AJ, Thomas J. Breast stimulation for cervical ripening and induction of labour. Cochrane Database Syst Rev. 2005 Jul 20;2005(3):CD003392. doi: 10.1002/14651858.CD003392.pub2

3. American College of Obstetricians and Gynecologists. First and second stage labor management (clinical practice guideline). 2024 Jan. **https://www.acog.org/clinical/clinical-guidance/clinical-practice-guideline/articles/2024/01/first-and-second-stage-labor-management**

WHO ARE THE PEOPLE WHO WILL BE CARING FOR ME ON LABOR AND DELIVERY?

1. Decesare JZ, Bush SY, Morton AN. Impact of an obstetrical hospitalist program on the safety events in a mid-sized obstetrical unit. J Patient Saf. 2020 Sep;16(3):e179–e181. doi: 10.1097/PTS.0000000000000397
2. Torbenson VE, Tatsis V, Bradley SL, Butler J, Kjerulff L, McLaughlin GB, Stika CS, Tappin D, VanBlaricom A, Mehta R, Branda M, McCue B. Use of obstetric and gynecologic hospitalists is associated with decreased severe maternal morbidity in the United States. J Patient Saf. 2023 Apr 1;19(3):202–210. doi: 10.1097/PTS.0000000000001102

WHAT IS NORMAL LABOR, ANYWAY?

1. American College of Obstetricians and Gynecologists. First and second stage labor management (clinical practice guideline). 2024 Jan. **https://www.acog.org/clinical/clinical-guidance/clinical-practice-guideline/articles/2024/01/first-and-second-stage-labor-management**

TALK TO ME ABOUT FETAL MONITORING.

1. American College of Obstetricians and Gynecologists. Intrapartum fetal heart rate monitoring: nomenclature, interpretation, and general management principles (practice bulletin). 2009 Jul. **https://www.acog.org/clinical/clinical-guidance/practice-bulletin/articles/2009/07/intrapartum-fetal-heart-rate-monitoring-nomenclature-interpretation-and-general-management-principles**
2. American College of Obstetricians and Gynecologists. Approaches to limit intervention during labor and birth (committee opinion). 2019 Feb; reaffirmed 2021. **https://www.acog.org/clinical/clinical-guidance/committee-opinion/articles/2019/02/approaches-to-limit-intervention-during-labor-and-birth**
3. Smith H, Peterson N, Lagrew D, Main E. 2016. Toolkit to Support Vaginal Birth and Reduce Primary Cesareans: A Quality Improvement Toolkit. Stanford, CA: California Maternal Quality Care Collaborative. **https://www.cmqcc.org/files/Vbirth-Toolkit-with-Supplement_Final_11.30.22_2.pdf**

AND THEY WANT TO PUT MONITORS . . . INSIDE OF ME?

1. American College of Obstetricians and Gynecologists. First and second stage labor management (clinical practice guideline). 2024 Jan. **https://www.acog.org/clinical/clinical-guidance/clinical-practice-guideline/articles/2024/01/first-and-second-stage-labor-management**
2. Kissler KJ, Lowe NK, Hernandez TL. An integrated review of uterine activity monitoring for evaluating labor dystocia. J Midwifery Womens Health. 2020 May;65(3):323–334. doi: 10.1111/jmwh.13119
3. Harper LM, Shanks AL, Tuuli MG, Roehl KA, Cahill AG. The risks and benefits of internal monitors in laboring patients. Am J Obstet Gynecol. 2013 Jul;209(1):38.e1–6. doi: 10.1016/j.ajog.2013.04.001
4. Liang Y, Li Y, Huang C, Li X, Cai Q, Peng J, Fan S. Safety of internal electronic fetal heart rate monitoring during labor. Matern Fetal Med. 2022 Mar 10;4(2):121–126. doi: 10.1097/FM9.0000000000000145
5. Kawakita T, Reddy UM, Landy HJ, Iqbal SN, Huang CC, Grantz KL. Neonatal complications associated with use of fetal scalp electrode: a retrospective study. BJOG. 2016 Oct;123(11):1797–803. doi: 10.1111/1471-0528.13817

CAN I EAT IN LABOR?

1. Sperling D, et al. Restriction of oral intake during labor: whither are we bound? Am J Obstet Gynecol. 2016 May;214(5):592–6. doi: 10.1016/j.ajog.2016.01.166
2. Singata M, Tranmer J, Gyte GML. Restricting oral fluid and food intake during labour. Cochrane Database Syst Rev. 2013 Aug 22;2013(8):CD003930. doi: 10.1002/14651858.CD003930.pub3
3. American Society of Anesthesiologists. Statement on oral intake during labor. 2022 Oct 26. **https://www.asahq.org/standards-and-practice-parameters/statement-on-oral-intake-during-labor**
4. American College of Obstetricians and Gynecologists. Approaches to limit intervention during labor and birth (committee opinion). 2019 Feb; reaffirmed 2021. **https://www.acog.org/clinical/clinical-guidance/committee-opinion/articles/2019/02/approaches-to-limit-intervention-during-labor-and-birth**
5. Yeo YH, Gaddam S, Ng WH, Huang PC, Motility and Metabolic Pharmacoepidemiology Group, Ma KS, Rezaie A. Increased risk of aspiration pneumonia associated with endoscopic procedures among patients with glucagon-like peptide 1 receptor agonist use. Gastroenterology. 2024 Jul;167(2):402–404.e3. doi: 10.1053/j.gastro.2024.03.015
6. Liew WJ, Negar A, Singh PA. Airway management in patients suffering from

morbid obesity. Saudi J Anaesth. 2022 Jul–Sep;16(3):314–321. doi: 10.4103/sja.sja_90_22

OW! I'M IN PAIN! WHAT CAN I DO?

1. American College of Obstetricians and Gynecologists. Obstetric analgesia and anesthesia (practice bulletin). 2019 Mar; reaffirmed 2024. **https://www.acog.org/clinical/clinical-guidance/practice-bulletin/articles/2019/03/obstetric-analgesia-and-anesthesia**
2. American College of Nurse Midwives. Position statement: hydrotherapy during labor and birth. 2022
3. Cluett ER, Burns E, Cuthbert A. Immersion in water during labour and birth. Cochrane Database Syst Rev. 2018 May 16;5(5):CD000111. doi: 10.1002/14651858.CD000111.pub4
4. Mårtensson LB, Hutton EK, Lee N, Kildea S, Gao Y, Bergh I. Sterile water injections for childbirth pain: an evidenced based guide to practice. Women Birth. 2018 Oct;31(5):380–385. **https://doi.org/10.1016/j.wombi.2017.12.001.**
5. Zuarez-Easton S, Erez O, Zafran N, Carmeli J, Garmi G, Salim R. Pharmacologic and nonpharmacologic options for pain relief during labor: an expert review. Am J Obstet Gynecol. 2023 May;228(5S):S1246–S1259. doi: 10.1016/j.ajog.2023.03.003
6. Bohren MA, Hofmeyr GJ, Sakala C, Fukuzawa RK, Cuthbert A. Continuous support for women during childbirth. Cochrane Database Syst Rev. 2017 Jul 6;7(7):CD003766. doi: 10.1002/14651858.CD003766.pub6

WHAT IS GETTING AN EPIDURAL LIKE?

1. American College of Obstetricians and Gynecologists. Obstetric analgesia and anesthesia (practice bulletin). 2019 Mar; reaffirmed 2024. **https://www.acog.org/clinical/clinical-guidance/practice-bulletin/articles/2019/03/obstetric-analgesia-and-anesthesia**
2. Anim-Somuah M, Smyth RM, Cyna AM, Cuthbert A. Epidural versus non-epidural or no analgesia for pain management in labour. Cochrane Database Syst Rev. 2018 May 21;5(5):CD000331. doi: 10.1002/14651858.CD000331.pub4
3. Pergialiotis V, Bellos I, Antsaklis A, Papapanagiotou A, Loutradis D, Daskalakis G. Maternal and neonatal outcomes following a prolonged second stage of labor: a meta-analysis of observational studies. Eur J Obstet Gynecol Reprod Biol. 2020 Sep;252:62–69. doi: 10.1016/j.ejogrb.2020.06.018
4. Akbas M, Akcan AB. Epidural analgesia and lactation. Eurasian J Med. 2011 Apr;43(1):45–9. doi: 10.5152/eajm.2011.09

5. American Society of Anesthesiologists. Statement on post-dural puncture headache management. 2021 Oct 13. **https://www.asahq.org/standards-and-practice-parameters/statement-on-post-dural-puncture-headache-management**
6. Thomas C, Banayan J. Do epidurals cause autism? (No.) A review of the controversy and what patients and providers need to know. Anesthesia Patient Safety Foundation. 2022 Feb. **https://www.apsf.org/article/do-epidurals-cause-autism-no-a-review-of-the-controversy-and-what-patients-and-providers-need-to-know**

WHAT IS THE BEST POSITION TO LABOR IN?

1. Lawrence A, Lewis L, Hofmeyr GJ, Styles C. Maternal positions and mobility during first stage labour. Cochrane Database Syst Rev. 2013 Aug 20;(8):CD003934. doi: 10.1002/14651858.CD003934.pub3. Update in: Cochrane Database Syst Rev. 2013 Oct 09;(10):CD003934. doi: 10.1002/14651858.CD003934.pub4
2. American College of Obstetricians and Gynecologists. Approaches to limit intervention during labor and birth (committee opinion). 2019 Feb; reaffirmed 2021. **https://www.acog.org/clinical/clinical-guidance/committee-opinion/articles/2019/02/approaches-to-limit-intervention-during-labor-and-birth**
3. American College of Obstetricians and Gynecologists. Approaches to limit intervention during labor and birth (committee opinion). 2019 Feb; reaffirmed 2021. **https://www.acog.org/clinical/clinical-guidance/committee-opinion/articles/2019/02/approaches-to-limit-intervention-during-labor-and-birth**
4. Cluett ER, Burns E, Cuthbert A. Immersion in water during labour and birth. Cochrane Database Syst Rev. 2018 May 16;5(5):CD000111. doi: 10.1002/14651858.CD000111.pub4

I WAS TOLD I'M GBS POSITIVE AND I'M FREAKING OUT.

1. American College of Obstetricians and Gynecologists. Prevention of group B streptococcal early-onset disease in newborns (committee opinion). 2020 Feb; reaffirmed 2022. **https://www.acog.org/clinical/clinical-guidance/committee-opinion/articles/2020/02/prevention-of-group-b-streptococcal-early-onset-disease-in-newborns**
2. Ohlsson A, Shah VS. Intrapartum antibiotics for known maternal Group B streptococcal colonization. Cochrane Database Syst Rev. 2014 Jun 10;(6):CD007467. doi: 10.1002/14651858.CD007467.pub4
3. Cutler RR, Odent M, Hajj-Ahmad H, Maharjan S, Bennett NJ, Josling PD,

Ball V, Hatton P, Dall'Antonia M. In vitro activity of an aqueous allicin extract and a novel allicin topical gel formulation against Lancefield group B streptococci. J Antimicrob Chemother. 2009 Jan;63(1):151–4. doi: 10.1093/jac/dkn457

4. Torres KAM, Lima SMRR, Torres LMB, Gamberini MT, Silva Jr PID. Garlic: an alternative treatment for group b streptococcus. Microbiol Spectr. 2021 Dec 22;9(3):e0017021. doi: 10.1128/Spectrum.00170-21
5. Hanson L, VandeVusse L, Malloy E, Garnier-Villarreal M, Watson L, Fial A, Forgie M, Nardini K, Safdar N. Probiotic interventions to reduce antepartum group B streptococcus colonization: a systematic review and meta-analysis. Midwifery. 2022 Feb;105:103208. doi: 10.1016/j.midw.2021.103208

MY DOCTOR WANTS TO BREAK MY BAG OF WATER AND I'M NOT SURE IF I SHOULD.

1. American College of Obstetricians and Gynecologists. First and second stage labor management (clinical practice guideline). 2024 Jan. **https://www.acog.org/clinical/clinical-guidance/clinical-practice-guideline/articles/2024/01/first-and-second-stage-labor-management**
2. American College of Obstetricians and Gynecologists. Approaches to limit intervention during labor and birth (committee opinion). 2019 Feb; reaffirmed 2021. **https://www.acog.org/clinical/clinical-guidance/committee-opinion/articles/2019/02/approaches-to-limit-intervention-during-labor-and-birth**
3. Kawakita T, Huang CC, Landy HJ. Risk factors for umbilical cord prolapse at the time of artificial rupture of membranes. AJP Rep. 2018 Apr;8(2):e89–e94. doi: 10.1055/s-0038-1649486

SHOULD I BE WORRIED ABOUT MECONIUM IN MY AMNIOTIC FLUID?

1. Chiruvolu A, Miklis KK, Chen E, Petrey B, Desai S. Delivery room management of meconium-stained newborns and respiratory support. Pediatrics. 2018 Dec;142(6):e20181485. doi: 10.1542/peds.2018-1485
2. American College of Obstetricians and Gynecologists. Delivery of a newborn with meconium-stained amniotic fluid (committee opinion). 2017 Mar; reaffirmed 2024. **https://www.acog.org/clinical/clinical-guidance/committee-opinion/articles/2017/03/delivery-of-a-newborn-with-meconium-stained-amniotic-fluid**
3. Osman A, Halling C, Crume M, Al Tabosh H, Odackal N, Ball MK. Meconium aspiration syndrome: a comprehensive review. J Perinatol. 2023 Oct;43(10):1211–1221. **https://doi.org/10.1038/s41372-023-01708-2**

4. Ward C, Caughey AB. The risk of meconium aspiration syndrome (MAS) increases with gestational age at term. J Matern Fetal Neonatal Med. 2022 Jan;35(1):155–160. **https://doi.org/10.1080/14767058.2020.1713744**

WHAT IS PITOCIN AND WHY MIGHT THEY SUGGEST I NEED IT?

1. Lothian JA. Healthy birth practice #4: avoid interventions unless they are medically necessary. J Perinat Educ. 2014 Fall;23(4):198–206. doi: 10.1891/1058-1243.23.4.198
2. American College of Obstetricians and Gynecologists. First and second stage labor management (clinical practice guideline). 2024 Jan. **https://www.acog.org/clinical/clinical-guidance/clinical-practice-guideline/articles/2024/01/first-and-second-stage-labor-management**
3. American College of Obstetricians and Gynecologists. Postpartum hemorrhage (practice bulletin). 2017 Oct. **https://www.acog.org/clinical/clinical-guidance/practice-bulletin/articles/2017/10/postpartum-hemorrhage**

THEY SAY MY LABOR IS GOING TOO SLOWLY— WHAT DOES THAT MEAN?

1. American College of Obstetricians and Gynecologists. Induction of labor (practice bulletin). 2009 Aug. **https://www.acog.org/clinical/clinical-guidance/practice-bulletin/articles/2009/08/induction-of-labor**
2. American College of Obstetricians and Gynecologists. First and second stage labor management (clinical practice guideline). 2024 Jan. **https://www.acog.org/clinical/clinical-guidance/clinical-practice-guideline/articles/2024/01/first-and-second-stage-labor-management**

TALK TO ME ABOUT C-SECTIONS.

1. Mackeen AD, Sullivan MV, Schuster M, Berghella V. Suture compared with staples for skin closure after cesarean delivery: a systematic review and meta-analysis. Obstet Gynecol. 2022 Aug 1;140(2):293–303. doi: 10.1097/AOG.0000000000004872
2. Dahlke JD, Mendez-Figueroa H, Maggio L, Sperling JD, Chauhan SP, Rouse DJ. The case for standardizing cesarean delivery technique: seeing the forest for the trees. Obstet Gynecol. 2020 Nov;136(5):972–980. doi: 10.1097/AOG.0000000000004120

WHAT AM I ALLOWED TO SAY NO TO?

1. Harp KLH, Bunting AM. The racialized nature of child welfare policies and the social control of black bodies. Soc Polit. 2020 Jun;27(2):258–281. doi: 10.1093/sp/jxz039

If Things Get Interesting

HELP, MY BABY IS BREECH! NOW WHAT?

1. American College of Obstetricians and Gynecologists. Mode of term singleton breech delivery (practice bulletin). 2018 Aug; reaffirmed 2023.
2. Coyle ME, Smith C, Peat B. Cephalic version by moxibustion for breech presentation. Cochrane Database Syst Rev. 2023 May 9;5(5):CD003928. doi: 10.1002/14651858.CD003928.pub4
3. Hofmeyr GJ, Kulier R. Cephalic version by postural management for breech presentation. Cochrane Database Syst Rev. 2012 Oct 17;10(10):CD000051. doi: 10.1002/14651858.CD000051.pub2
4. Kim GJ. Reviving external cephalic version: a review of its efficacy, safety, and technical aspects. Obstet Gynecol Sci. 2019 Nov;62(6):371–381. doi: 10.5468/ogs.2019.62.6.371
5. Goetzinger KR, Harper LM, Tuuli MG, Macones GA, Colditz GA. Effect of regional anesthesia on the success rate of external cephalic version: a systematic review and meta-analysis. Obstet Gynecol. 2011 Nov;118(5):1137–1144. doi: 10.1097/AOG.0b013e3182324583

I WAS TOLD I HAVE HIGH BLOOD PRESSURE AND I'M SCARED.

1. American College of Obstetricians and Gynecologists. Gestational hypertension and preeclampsia (practice bulletin). 2020 Jun. **https://www.acog.org/clinical/clinical-guidance/practice-bulletin/articles/2020/06/gestational-hypertension-and-preeclampsia**
2. American College of Obstetricians and Gynecologists. Chronic hypertension in pregnancy (practice bulletin). 2019 Jan. **https://www.acog.org/clinical/clinical-guidance/practice-bulletin/articles/2019/01/chronic-hypertension-in-pregnancy**
3. American College of Obstetricians and Gynecologists. Medically indicated late preterm and early-term deliveries (committee opinion). 2021 Jul. **https://www.acog.org/clinical/clinical-guidance/committee-opinion/articles/2021/07/medically-indicated-late-preterm-and-early-term-deliveries**

I'VE STARTED BLEEDING TOO MUCH—WHAT'S GOING ON?

1. Brandt JS, Ananth CV. Placental abruption at near-term and term gestations: pathophysiology, epidemiology, diagnosis, and management. Am J Obstet Gynecol. 2023 May;228(5S):S1313–S1329. doi: 10.1016/j.ajog.2022.06.059
2. American College of Obstetricians and Gynecologists. Postpartum hemorrhage (practice bulletin). 2017 Oct. **https://www.acog.org/clinical/clinical-guidance/practice-bulletin/articles/2017/10/postpartum-hemorrhage**
3. D'Alton ME, Rood KM, Smid MC, Simhan HN, Skupski DW, Subramaniam A, Gibson KS, Rosen T, Clark SM, Dudley D, Iqbal SN, Paglia MJ, Duzyj CM, Chien EK, Gibbins KJ, Wine KD, Bentum NAA, Kominiarek MA, Tuuli MG, Goffman D. Intrauterine vacuum-induced hemorrhage-control device for rapid treatment of postpartum hemorrhage. Obstet Gynecol. 2020 Nov;136(5):882–891. doi: 10.1097/AOG.0000000000004138

WHAT IS A SHOULDER DYSTOCIA?

1. American College of Obstetricians and Gynecologists. Shoulder dystocia (practice bulletin). 2017 May. **https://www.acog.org/clinical/clinical-guidance/practice-bulletin/articles/2017/05/shoulder-dystocia**

WHY DO I HAVE A FEVER IN LABOR?

1. Patel S, Ciechanowicz S, Blumenfeld YJ, Sultan P. Epidural-related maternal fever: incidence, pathophysiology, outcomes, and management. Am J Obstet Gynecol. 2023 May;228(5S):S1283–S1304.e1. **https://www.ajog.org/article/S0002-9378(22)00480-X/pdf**
2. American College of Obstetricians and Gynecologists. Intrapartum management of intraamniotic infection (committee opinion). 2017 Aug; reaffirmed 2022. **https://www.acog.org/clinical/clinical-guidance/committee-opinion/articles/2017/08/intrapartum-management-of-intraamniotic-infection**

The Grand Entrance (or Exit)

MY NURSE SAYS IT'S TIME TO PUSH. HELP!

1. American College of Obstetricians and Gynecologists. Approaches to limit intervention during labor and birth (committee opinion). 2019 Feb; reaffirmed 2021. **https://www.acog.org/clinical/clinical-guidance/committee-opinion/articles/2019/02/approaches-to-limit-intervention-during-labor-and-birth**

WHAT IS THE BEST POSITION TO PUSH AND DELIVER MY BABY IN?

1. Gupta JK, Sood A, Hofmeyr GJ, Vogel JP. Position in the second stage of labour for women without epidural anaesthesia. Cochrane Database Syst Rev. 2017 May 25;5(5):CD002006. doi: 10.1002/14651858.CD002006.pub4
2. Kibuka M, Thornton JG. Position in the second stage of labour for women with epidural anaesthesia. Cochrane Database Syst Rev. 2017 Feb 24;2(2):CD008070. doi: 10.1002/14651858.CD008070.pub3. Update in: Cochrane Database Syst Rev. 2018 Nov 09;11:CD008070. doi: 10.1002/14651858.CD008070.pub4
3. Zang Y, Lu H, Zhao Y, Huang J, Ren L, Li X. Effects of flexible sacrum positions during the second stage of labour on maternal and neonatal outcomes: a systematic review and meta-analysis. J Clin Nurs. 2020 Sep;29(17–18):3154–3169. doi: 10.1111/jocn.15376
4. Upright versus lying down position in second stage of labour in nulliparous women with low dose epidural: BUMPES randomised controlled trial. BMJ. 2017;359:j4471. doi:10.1136/bmj.j4471
5. World Health Organization. WHO recommends intrapartum care for a positive childbirth experience. 2018. **https://iris.who.int/bitstream/handle/10665/272447/WHO-RHR-18.12-eng.pdf**
6. American College of Obstetricians and Gynecologists. Approaches to limit intervention during labor and birth (committee opinion). 2019 Feb; reaffirmed 2021. **https://www.acog.org/clinical/clinical-guidance/committee-opinion/articles/2019/02/approaches-to-limit-intervention-during-labor-and-birth**
7. American College of Nurse-Midwives, Midwives Alliance of North America, National Association of Certified Professional Midwives. Supporting healthy and normal physiologic childbirth: a consensus statement by the American College of Nurse-Midwives, Midwives Alliance of North America, and the National Association of Certified Professional Midwives. J Midwifery Womens Health. 2012 Sep–Oct;57(5):529–32. doi: 10.1111/j.1542-2011.2012.00218.x
8. Simpson KR, Creehan PA, O'Brien-Abel N, et al. Perinatal Nursing, 5e. 2021; Lippincott Williams & Wilkins. **https://advisor.lwwhealthlibrary.com/book.aspx?bookid=3096§ionid=0.**
9. Association of Women's Health, Obstetric, and Neonatal Nurses. Nursing care and management of the second stage of labor: evidence-based clinical practice guideline. Third ed. 2019. **https://search.ebscohost.com/login.aspx?direct=true&scope=site&db=nlebk&db=nlabk&AN=2367265**

HOW LONG IS PUSHING GOING TO TAKE?

1. American College of Obstetricians and Gynecologists. First and second stage labor management (clinical practice guideline). 2024 Jan. **https://www.acog.org/clinical/clinical-guidance/clinical-practice-guideline/articles/2024/01/first-and-second-stage-labor-management**
2. Cheng YW, Shaffer BL, Nicholson JM, Caughey AB. Second stage of labor and epidural use: a larger effect than previously suggested. Obstet Gynecol. 2014 Mar;123(3):527–535. doi: 10.1097/AOG.0000000000000134. Erratum in: Obstet Gynecol. 2014 May;123(5):1109

THEY'RE TELLING ME I NEED A C-SECTION BUT I DON'T THINK I NEED ONE. CAN I SAY NO?

1. American College of Obstetricians and Gynecologists. Macrosomia (practice bulletin). 2020 Jan. **https://www.acog.org/clinical/clinical-guidance/practice-bulletin/articles/2020/01/macrosomia**

WHAT IS A VACUUM OR FORCEPS, AND WHY MIGHT I NEED IT?

1. American College of Obstetricians and Gynecologists. Operative vaginal birth (practice bulletin). 2020 Apr; reaffirmed 2021.
2. Gyhagen M, Bullarbo M, Nielsen TF, Milsom I. Prevalence and risk factors for pelvic organ prolapse 20 years after childbirth: a national cohort study in singleton primiparae after vaginal or caesarean delivery. BJOG. 2013 Jan;120(2):152–160. doi: 10.1111/1471-0528.12020
3. Handa VL, Blomquist JL, McDermott KC, Friedman S, Muñoz A. Pelvic floor disorders after vaginal birth: effect of episiotomy, perineal laceration, and operative birth. Obstet Gynecol. 2012 Feb;119(2 Pt 1):233–9. doi: 10.1097/AOG.0b013e318240df4f
4. Memon HU, Blomquist JL, Dietz HP, Pierce CB, Weinstein MM, Handa VL. Comparison of levator ani muscle avulsion injury after forceps-assisted and vacuum-assisted vaginal childbirth. Obstet Gynecol. 2015 May;125(5):1080–1087. doi: 10.1097/AOG.0000000000000825
5. Blomquist JL, Muñoz A, Carroll M, Handa VL. Association of delivery mode with pelvic floor disorders after childbirth. JAMA. 2018;320(23):2438–2447. doi:10.1001/jama.2018.18315
6. Arya LA, Jackson ND, Myers DL, Verma A. Risk of new-onset urinary incontinence after forceps and vacuum delivery in primiparous women. Am J

Obstet Gynecol. 2001 Dec;185(6):1318–23; discussion 1323–4. doi: 10.1067/mob.2001.120365

7. Blomquist JL, McDermott K, Handa VL. Pelvic pain and mode of delivery. Am J Obstet Gynecol. 2014 May;210(5):423.e1–6. doi: 10.1016/j.ajog.2014.01.032
8. Duval M, Daniel SJ. Facial nerve palsy in neonates secondary to forceps use. Arch Otolaryngol Head Neck Surg. 2009;135(7):634–636. doi:10.1001/archoto.2009.69
9. StatPearls. Birth trauma. **https://www.statpearls.com/ArticleLibrary/viewarticle/18338**

MY BABY IS "SUNNY SIDE UP" AND I AM NOT SURE WHAT THAT MEANS.

1. American College of Obstetricians and Gynecologists. First and second stage labor management (clinical practice guideline). 2024 Jan. **https://www.acog.org/clinical/clinical-guidance/clinical-practice-guideline/articles/2024/01/first-and-second-stage-labor-management**
2. Bahmaei H, Mousavi P, Haghighizadeh MH, Iravani M. The impact of maternal position in labor on occiput-posterior position of fetus and pregnancy outcomes in pregnant women without epidural analgesia. J Family Reprod Health. 2023 Jun;17(2):86–92. doi: 10.18502/jfrh.v17i2.12871

HOW DO I PREVENT TEARING?

1. American College of Obstetricians and Gynecologists. Prevention and management of obstetric lacerations at vaginal delivery (practice bulletin). 2018 Sep; reaffirmed 2022. **https://www.acog.org/clinical/clinical-guidance/practice-bulletin/articles/2018/09/prevention-and-management-of-obstetric-lacerations-at-vaginal-delivery**
2. Sandall J, Fernandez Turienzo C, Devane D, Soltani H, Gillespie P, Gates S, Jones LV, Shennan AH, Rayment-Jones H. Midwife continuity of care models versus other models of care for childbearing women. Cochrane Database Syst Rev. 2024 Apr 10;4(4):CD004667. doi: 10.1002/14651858.CD004667.pub6

WILL I NEED AN EPISIOTOMY?

1. Leapfrog Group. State of maternity care in the U.S.: the Leapfrog Group 2023 report on trends in C-sections, early elective deliveries, and episiotomies. 2023. **https://www.leapfroggroup.org/sites/default/files/Files/2023%20Maternity%20Report_Final_0.pdf**

2. American College of Obstetricians and Gynecologists. Prevention and management of obstetric lacerations at vaginal delivery (practice bulletin). 2018 Sep; reaffirmed 2022. **https://www.acog.org/clinical/clinical-guidance/practice-bulletin/articles/2018/09/prevention-and-management-of-obstetric-lacerations-at-vaginal-delivery**
3. Leapfrog Group. Episiotomy rates from the 2015 Leapfrog hospital survey. **https://www.leapfroggroup.org/sites/default/files/Files/2015_MaternityCareData_Episiotomy.pdf**
4. Leapfrog Group. Search Leapfrog's hospital and surgery center ratings. **https://ratings.leapfroggroup.org**

WHAT HAPPENS WHEN THE BABY COMES OUT?

1. Hammer NC, Koch JJ, Hopkins HC. Neonatal resuscitation: updated guidelines from the American Heart Association. Am Fam Physician. 2021 Oct 1;104(4):425–428
2. Lazzeri J, Giordano NA, Christ L, Polomano RC, Stringer M. Hats off for full-term healthy newborns: no benefits for thermoregulation. J Perinat Neonatal Nurs. 2023 Oct–Dec 01;37(4):340–347. doi: 10.1097/JPN.0000000000000758
3. Lundström JN, Mathe A, Schaal B, Frasnelli J, Nitzsche K, Gerber J, Hummel T. Maternal status regulates cortical responses to the body odor of newborns. Front Psychol. 2013 Sep 5;4:597. **https://www.frontiersin.org/journals/psychology/articles/10.3389/fpsyg.2013.00597/full**

SHOULD I ASK FOR DELAYED CORD CLAMPING?

1. American College of Obstetricians and Gynecologists. Delayed umbilical cord clamping after birth (committee opinion). 2020 Dec; reaffirmed 2023. **https://www.acog.org/clinical/clinical-guidance/committee-opinion/articles/2020/12/delayed-umbilical-cord-clamping-after-birth**

SHOULD I BANK MY BABY'S CORD BLOOD?

1. American College of Obstetricians and Gynecologists. Umbilical cord blood banking (committee opinion). 2019 Mar; reaffirmed 2023. **https://www.acog.org/clinical/clinical-guidance/committee-opinion/articles/2019/03/umbilical-cord-blood-banking**
2. NMDP. Public cord blood banks and donation hospitals. **https://www.nmdp.org/what-we-do/partnerships/global-transplant-network/cord-blood-banks-and-hospitals**

WHEN (AND HOW) DOES THE PLACENTA COME OUT?

1. American College of Obstetricians and Gynecologists. Postpartum hemorrhage (practice bulletin). 2017 Oct. **https://www.acog.org/clinical/clinical-guidance/practice-bulletin/articles/2017/10/postpartum-hemorrhage**
2. Hersh AR, Carroli G, Hofmeyr GJ, Garg B, Gülmezoglu M, Lumbiganon P, De Mucio B, Saleem S, Festin MPR, Mittal S, Rubio-Romero JA, Chipato T, Valencia C, Tolosa JE. Third stage of labor: evidence-based practice for prevention of adverse maternal and neonatal outcomes. Am J Obstet Gynecol. 2024 Mar;230(3S):S1046–S1060.e1. doi: 10.1016/j.ajog.2022.11.1298

SHOULD I TAKE MY PLACENTA HOME?

1. Buser GL, Mató S, Zhang AY, Metcalf BJ, Beall B, Thomas AR. Notes from the field: late-onset infant group B streptococcus infection associated with maternal consumption of capsules containing dehydrated placenta—Oregon, 2016. MMWR Morb Mortal Wkly Rep 2017;66:677–678. **http://dx.doi.org/10.15585/mmwr.mm6625a4**
2. Benyshek DC, Bovbjerg ML, Cheyney M. Comparison of placenta consumers' and non-consumers' postpartum depression screening results using EPDS in US community birth settings (n=6038): a propensity score analysis. BMC Pregnancy Childbirth. 2023 Jul 22;23(1):534. **https://doi.org/10.1186/s12884-023-05852-7**
3. Kyejo W, Rubagumya D, Mwalo C, Moshi L, Kaguta M, Mgonja M, Jaiswal S. "Do not detach the placenta from my baby's cord"—lotus birth case series from Tanzania tertiary hospital. Int J Surg Case Rep. 2022 Oct;99:107630. doi: 10.1016/j.ijscr.2022.107630

WHAT IS THIS "GOLDEN HOUR" I KEEP HEARING ABOUT?

1. Moore ER, Bergman N, Anderson GC, Medley N. Early skin-to-skin contact for mothers and their healthy newborn infants. Cochrane Database Syst Rev. 2012 May 16;5(5):CD003519. doi: 10.1002/14651858.CD003519.pub3. Update in: Cochrane Database Syst Rev. 2016 Nov 25;11:CD003519. doi: 10.1002/14651858.CD003519.pub4
2. Gouchon S, Gregori D, Picotto A, Patrucco G, Nangeroni M, Di Giulio P. Skin-to-skin contact after cesarean delivery: an experimental study. Nurs Res. 2010 Mar–Apr;59(2):78–84. doi: 10.1097/NNR.0b013e3181d1a8bc

CAN I HAVE AN IUD PLACED RIGHT AFTER I HAVE MY BABY?

1. American College of Obstetricians and Gynecologists. Long-acting reversible contraception implants and intrauterine devices (practice bulletin). 2017 Nov. **https://www.acog.org/clinical/clinical-guidance/practice-bulletin/articles/2017/11/long-acting-reversible-contraception-implants-and-intrauterine-devices**
2. American College of Obstetricians and Gynecologists. Optimizing postpartum care (committee opinion). 2018 May; reaffirmed 2021. **https://www.acog.org/clinical/clinical-guidance/committee-opinion/articles/2018/05/optimizing-postpartum-care**

CAN YOU EXPLAIN WHY MY BABY GETS SHOTS AND EYE OINTMENT WHEN THEY'RE BORN?

1. Hand I, Noble L, Abrams SA. Vitamin K and the newborn infant. Pediatrics. 2022 Mar 1;149(3):e2021056036. doi: 10.1542/peds.2021-056036
2. Children's Hospital of Philadelphia. Hepatitis B: the disease and vaccines. **https://www.chop.edu/vaccine-education-center/vaccine-details/hepatitis-b-vaccine**
3. Hand I, Noble L, Abrams SA. Vitamin K and the newborn infant. Pediatrics. 2022 Mar 1;149(3):e2021056036. doi: 10.1542/peds.2021-056036
4. Centers for Disease Control and Prevention. Frequently asked questions about vitamin K deficiency bleeding. 2025 Jan 17. **https://www.cdc.gov/vitamin-k-deficiency/faq**
5. Koklu E, Taskale T, Koklu S, Ariguloglu EA. Anaphylactic shock due to vitamin K in a newborn and review of literature. J Matern Fetal Neonatal Med. 2014 Jul;27(11):1180–1. doi: 10.3109/14767058.2013.847425
6. Britt RB, Brown JN. Characterizing the severe reactions of parenteral vitamin K1. Clin Appl Thromb Hemost. 2018 Jan;24(1):5–12. doi: 10.1177/1076029616674825
7. World Health Organization. Hepatitis B. 2024 Apr 9. **https://www.who.int/news-room/fact-sheets/detail/hepatitis-b**
8. New York State Department of Health. Every week hundreds of people get hepatitis B. 2012 Oct. **https://www.health.ny.gov/publications/2340**
9. Children's Hospital of Philadelphia. Hepatitis B: what you should know. 2022 Summer. **https://www.chop.edu/sites/default/files/vaccine-education-center-hepatitis-b.pdf**

CAN THEY BATHE MY BABY BEFORE I HOLD THEM?

1. Priyadarshi M, Balachander B, Gupta S, Sankar MJ. Timing of first bath in term healthy newborns: a systematic review. J Glob Health. 2022 Aug 17;12:12004. doi: 10.7189/jogh.12.12004
2. Kirts E, Shell T, International Childbirth Education Association (ICEA). Delayed bathing: position paper. ICEA. **https://icea.org/wp-content/uploads/2022/09/ICEA-Position-Paper-Delayed-Bathing.pdf**

The Afterparty

WHERE DOES MY BABY STAY?

1. Feldman-Winter L, Goldsmith JP, Committee on Fetus and Newborn, Task Force on Sudden Infant Death Syndrome. Safe sleep and skin-to-skin care in the neonatal period for healthy term newborns. Pediatrics. 2016 Sep;138(3):e20161889. **https://publications.aap.org/pediatrics/article/doi/10.1542/peds.2016-1889/52741/Safe-Sleep-and-Skin-to-Skin-Care-in-the-Neonatal**
2. Theo LO, Drake E. Rooming-in: creating a better experience. J Perinat Educ. 2017;26(2):79–84. doi: 10.1891/1058-1243.26.2.79

WHAT DO I DO FOR PAIN?

1. American College of Obstetricians and Gynecologists. Pharmacologic stepwise multimodal approach for postpartum pain management (clinical consensus). 2021 Sep. **https://www.acog.org/clinical/clinical-guidance/clinical-consensus/articles/2021/09/pharmacologic-stepwise-multimodal-approach-for-postpartum-pain-management**
2. de Queiroz VKP, da Nóbrega Marinho AM, de Barros GAM. Analgesic effects of a 5% lidocaine patch after cesarean section: a randomized placebo-controlled double-blind clinical trial. J Clin Anesth. 2021 Oct;73:110328. doi: 10.1016/j.jclinane.2021.110328
3. U.S. Food and Drug Administration. Use of codeine and tramadol products in breastfeeding women—questions and answers. 2019 Aug 1. **https://www.fda.gov/drugs/postmarket-drug-safety-information-patients-and-providers/use-codeine-and-tramadol-products-breastfeeding-women-questions-and-answers**

WHO CAN HELP ME WITH BREASTFEEDING?

1. US Lactation Consultants Association. Who's who? A glance at breastfeeding support in the United States. **https://uslca.org/wp-content/uploads/2016/06/2-page-Whos-Who.pdf**

I DON'T WANT TO BREASTFEED, SO WHAT SHOULD I DO?

1. Oladapo OT, Fawole B. Treatments for suppression of lactation. Cochrane Database Syst Rev. 2012 Sep 12;2012(9):CD005937. doi: 10.1002/14651858.CD005937.pub3
2. Henkel A, Johnson SA, Reeves MF, Cahill EP, Blumenthal PD, Shaw KA. Cabergoline for lactation inhibition after second-trimester abortion or pregnancy loss: a randomized controlled trial. Obstet Gynecol. 2023 Jun 1;141(6):1115–1123. **https://journals.lww.com/greenjournal/fulltext/2023/06000/cabergoline_for_lactation_inhibition_after.11.aspx**
3. Yang Y, Boucoiran I, Tulloch KJ, Poliquin V. Is cabergoline safe and effective for postpartum lactation inhibition? A systematic review. Int J Womens Health. 2020 Mar 9;12:159–170. doi: 10.2147/IJWH.S232693
4. Johnson HM, Eglash A, Mitchell KB, Leeper K, Smillie CM, Moore-Ostby L, Manson N, Simon L, Academy of Breastfeeding Medicine. ABM clinical protocol #32: management of hyperlactation. Breastfeed Med. 2020 Mar;15(3):129–134. **https://www.bfmed.org/assets/DOCUMENTS/PROTOCOLS/Protocol%20%2332%20-%20English%20Translation.pdf**
5. Boi B, Koh S, Gail D. The effectiveness of cabbage leaf application (treatment) on pain and hardness in breast engorgement and its effect on the duration of breastfeeding. JBI Libr Syst Rev. 2012;10(20):1185–1213. doi: 10.11124/01938924-201210200-00001
6. Drugs and Lactation Database (LactMed). 2006. **https://www.ncbi.nlm.nih.gov/books/NBK501774**
7. Aljazaf K, Hale TW, Ilett KF, Hartmann PE, Mitoulas LR, Kristensen JH, Hackett LP. Pseudoephedrine: effects on milk production in women and estimation of infant exposure via breastmilk. Br J Clin Pharmacol. 2003 Jul;56(1):18–24. doi: 10.1046/j.1365-2125.2003.01822.x

SHOULD I DO VAGINAL SEEDING IF I'VE HAD A C-SECTION?

1. American College of Obstetricians and Gynecologists. Vaginal seeding (committee opinion). 2017 Nov; reaffirmed 2025. **https://www.acog.org/clinical/clinical-guidance/committee-opinion/articles/2017/11/vaginal-seeding**

2. Nolt D, O'Leary ST, Aucott SW, Committee on Infectious Diseases and Committee on Fetus and Newborn. Risks of infectious diseases in newborns exposed to alternative perinatal practices. Pediatrics. 2022 Feb 1;149(2):e2021055554. doi: 10.1542/peds.2021-055554

WHAT DO I NEED TO KNOW ABOUT TONGUE TIE?

1. LeFort Y, Evans A, Livingstone V, Douglas P, Dahlquist N, Donnelly B, Leeper K, Harley E, Lappin S. Academy of Breastfeeding Medicine position statement on ankyloglossia in breastfeeding dyads. Breastfeed Med. 2021 Apr;16(4):278–281. **https://www.bfmed.org/assets/Anklyloglossia%20position%20statement%202021.pdf**
2. Thomas J, Bunik M, Holmes A, Keels MA, Poindexter B, Meyer A, Gilliland A, Section on Breastfeeding, Section on Oral Health, Council on Quality Improvement and Patient Safety, Committee on Fetus and Newborn, Section on Otolaryngology-Head and Neck Surgery. Identification and management of ankyloglossia and its effect on breastfeeding in infants: clinical report. Pediatrics August 2024; 154 (2): e2024067605. 10.1542/peds.2024-067605
3. McKechnie AC, Eglash A. Nipple shields: a review of the literature. Breastfeed Med. 2010 Dec;5(6):309–14. doi: 10.1089/bfm.2010.0003
4. Coentro VS, Perrella SL, Lai CT, Rea A, Murray K, Geddes DT. Effect of nipple shield use on milk removal: a mechanistic study. 2020 Sep 7;20(1):516. https://doi.org/10.1186/s12884-020-03191-5

WHAT'S UP WITH CIRCUMCISION, AND WHO DO I ASK?

1. American Association of Pediatrics. Should the baby be circumcised? 2024 Feb 12. **https://www.healthychildren.org/English/ages-stages/prenatal/decisions-to-make/Pages/Should-the-Baby-be-Circumcised.aspx**
2. Jacobson DL, Balmert LC, Holl JL, Rosoklija I, Davis MM, Johnson EK. Nationwide circumcision trends: 2003 to 2016. J Urol. 2021 Jan;205(1):257–263. doi: 10.1097/JU.0000000000001316
3. Morris BJ, Wamai RG, Henebeng EB, Tobian AA, Klausner JD, Banerjee J, Hankins CA. Estimation of country-specific and global prevalence of male circumcision. Popul Health Metr. 2016 Mar 1;14:4. doi: 10.1186/s12963-016-0073-5. Erratum in: Popul Health Metr. 2016 Apr 04;14:11. doi: 10.1186/s12963-016-0080-6
4. Theoharakis M, Feldman E, Friedman S. Circumcision. Pediatr Rev. 2022 Dec 1;43(12):728–730. **https://doi.org/10.1542/pir.2022-005536**

5. Centers for Disease Control and Prevention, National Center for Health Statistics. Trends in circumcision for male newborns in U.S. hospitals: 1979–2010. **https://www.cdc.gov/nchs/data/hestat/circumcision_2013/circumcision_2013.htm#national_trends**

I AM TERRIFIED TO POOP.

1. Short V, Herbert G, Perry R, Atkinson C, Ness AR, Penfold C, Thomas S, Andersen HK, Lewis SJ. Chewing gum for postoperative recovery of gastrointestinal function. Cochrane Database Syst Rev. 2015 Feb 20;2015(2):CD006506. doi: 10.1002/14651858.CD006506.pub3
2. Paauw D. Myth of the month: does Colace work? MD Edge. 2015 Nov 19. **https://www.mdedge.com/familymedicine/article/104548/gastroenterology/myth-month-does-colace-work**
3. Rao SSC, Brenner DM. Efficacy and safety of over-the-counter therapies for chronic constipation: an updated systematic review. Am J Gastroenterol. 2021 Jun 1;116(6):1156–1181. doi: 10.14309/ajg.0000000000001222

WHAT IS THE BIRTH CONTROL SITUATION?

1. Abebe Gelaw K, Atalay YA, Yeshambel A, Adella GA, Walle BG, Zeleke LB, Gebeyehu NA. Prevalence and factors associated with early resumption of sexual intercourse among postpartum women: systematic review and meta-analysis. PLoS One. 2024 Jan 17;19(1):e0288536. doi: 10.1371/journal.pone.0288536
2. Curtis KM, Tepper NK, Jatlaoui TC, et al. U.S. medical eligibility criteria for contraceptive use, 2016. MMWR Recomm Rep 2016;65(No. RR-3):1–104. **http://dx.doi.org/10.15585/mmwr.rr6503a1**
3. Berens P, Labbok M, Academy of Breastfeeding Medicine. ABM clinical protocol #13: contraception during breastfeeding, revised 2015. Breastfeed Med. 2015 Jan–Feb;10(1):3–12. **https://www.bfmed.org/assets/DOCUMENTS/PROTOCOLS/13-contraception-and-breastfeeding-protocol-english.pdf**
4. Curtis KM, Nguyen AT, Tepper NK, et al. U.S. selected practice recommendations for contraceptive use, 2024. MMWR Recomm Rep 2024;73(No. RR-3):1–77. **http://dx.doi.org/10.15585/mmwr.rr6503a1**
5. GoodRx. Slynd. **https://www.goodrx.com/slynd/what-is**
6. Bedsider website. **www.bedsider.org**

I FORGOT ALL THE DISCHARGE INSTRUCTIONS SO . . . CAN YOU REPEAT THEM?

1. American College of Obstetricians and Gynecologists. Exercise after pregnancy. FAQ131. 2024 Oct. **https://www.acog.org/womens-health/faqs/exercise-after-pregnancy**
2. U.S. Department of Health and Human Services. Move your way. **https://health.gov/moveyourway#during-after-pregnancy**
3. American College of Obstetricians and Gynecologists. Physical activity and exercise during pregnancy and the postpartum period (committee opinion). 2020 Apr; reaffirmed 2023. **https://www.acog.org/clinical/clinical-guidance/committee-opinion/articles/2020/04/physical-activity-and-exercise-during-pregnancy-and-the-postpartum-period**
4. Shirah BH, Shirah HA, Fallata AH, Alobidy SN, Hawsawi MMA. Hemorrhoids during pregnancy: sitz bath vs. ano-rectal cream: a comparative prospective study of two conservative treatment protocols. Women Birth. 2018 Aug;31(4):e272–e277. doi: 10.1016/j.wombi.2017.10.003
5. American College of Obstetricians and Gynecologists. Gestational hypertension and preeclampsia (practice bulletin). 2020 Jun. **https://www.acog.org/clinical/clinical-guidance/practice-bulletin/articles/2020/06/gestational-hypertension-and-preeclampsia**
6. American College of Obstetricians and Gynecologists. Optimizing postpartum care (committee opinion). 2018 May; reaffirmed 2021. **https://www.acog.org/clinical/clinical-guidance/committee-opinion/articles/2018/05/optimizing-postpartum-care**
7. Kealy MA, Small RE, Liamputtong P. Recovery after caesarean birth: a qualitative study of women's accounts in Victoria, Australia. BMC Pregnancy Childbirth. 2010 Aug 18;10:47. doi: 10.1186/1471-2393-10-47

WHAT DO I DO IF I THINK I HAVE POSTPARTUM DEPRESSION OR ANXIETY?

1. American College of Obstetricians and Gynecologists. Treatment and management of mental health conditions during pregnancy and postpartum (clinical practice guideline). 2023 Jun. **https://www.acog.org/clinical/clinical-guidance/clinical-practice-guideline/articles/2023/06/treatment-and-management-of-mental-health-conditions-during-pregnancy-and-postpartum**
2. American College of Obstetricians and Gynecologists. Screening and diagnosis of mental health conditions during pregnancy and postpartum (clinical practice guideline). 2023 Jun. **https://www.acog.org/clinical/clinical-guidance/**

clinical-practice-guideline/articles/2023/06/screening-and-diagnosis-of-mental-health-conditions-during-pregnancy-and-postpartum

3. Johns Hopkins Medicine. Baby blues and postpartum depression: mood disorders and pregnancy. **https://www.hopkinsmedicine.org/health/wellness-and-prevention/postpartum-mood-disorders-what-new-moms-need-to-know**
4. Nakić Radoš S, Tadinac M, Herman R. Anxiety during pregnancy and postpartum: course, predictors and comorbidity with postpartum depression. Acta Clin Croat. 2018 Mar;57(1):39–51. doi: 10.20471/acc.2017.56.04.05

I THINK I HAD A TRAUMATIC BIRTH AND I DON'T KNOW WHERE TO GO FOR HELP.

1. Maternal Mental Health Leadership Alliance. Birth trauma and maternal mental health. 2023 Aug. **https://static1.squarespace.com/static/637b72cb2e3c555fa412eaf0/t/66cdb018b52c946a990ee1e7/1724755998893/FINAL+VERSION+-+Birth+Trauma+Fact+Sheet.pdf**
2. American College of Obstetricians and Gynecologists. Caring for patients who have experienced trauma (committee opinion). 2021 Apr; reaffirmed 2024. **https://www.acog.org/clinical/clinical-guidance/committee-opinion/articles/2021/04/caring-for-patients-who-have-experienced-trauma**
3. World Health Organization. The prevention and elimination of disrespect and abuse during facility-based childbirth. 2015. **https://iris.who.int/bitstream/handle/10665/134588/WHO_RHR_14.23_eng.pdf;jsessionid=8E5A99EF961C01DF6B76DCC0D80B798E?sequence=1**
4. Chervenak FA, McLeod-Sordjan R, Pollet SL, De Four Jones M, Gordon MR, Combs A, Bornstein E, Lewis D, Katz A, Warman A, Grünebaum A. Obstetric violence is a misnomer. Am J Obstet Gynecol. 2024 Mar;230(3S):S1138–S1145. doi: 10.1016/j.ajog.2023.10.003
5. Make Birth Better website. **https://www.makebirthbetter.org**
6. Postpartum Support International. PSI online support meetings. **https://www.postpartum.net/get-help/psi-online-support-meetings**
7. Birth Trauma Association website. **https://www.birthtraumaassociation.org**

IS EVERYTHING NORMAL DOWN THERE? BECAUSE IT DOESN'T FEEL THAT WAY . . .

1. American College of Obstetricians and Gynecologists. Urinary incontinence in women (practice bulletin). 2015 Nov. **https://www.acog.org/clinical/clinical-guidance/practice-bulletin/articles/2015/11/urinary-incontinence-in-women**

Stillbirth

WHAT ARE MY OPTIONS FOR DELIVERY?

1. Boyle A, Preslar JP, Hogue CJ, Silver RM, Reddy UM, Goldenberg RL, Stoll BJ, Varner MW, Conway DL, Saade GR, Bukowski R, Dudley DJ. Route of delivery in women with stillbirth: results from the Stillbirth Collaborative Research Network. Obstet Gynecol. 2017 Apr;129(4):693–698. doi: 10.1097/AOG.0000000000001935
2. Burden C, Merriel A, Bakhbakhi D, Heazell A, Siassakos D; Royal College of Obstetricians and Gynaecologists. Care of late intrauterine fetal death and stillbirth: green-top guideline no. 55. BJOG. 2025 Jan;132(1):e1–e41. **https://doi.org/10.1111/1471-0528.17844**
3. American College of Obstetricians and Gynecologists. Management of stillbirth (obstetric care consensus). 2020 Mar. **https://www.acog.org/clinical/clinical-guidance/obstetric-care-consensus/articles/2020/03/management-of-stillbirth**

WHAT CAUSED THIS?

1. Centers for Disease Control and Prevention. Talking with families about stillbirth. 2024 Oct 24. **https://www.cdc.gov/stillbirth/hcp/conversation-tips/index.html**
2. American College of Obstetricians and Gynecologists. Management of stillbirth (obstetric care consensus). 2020 Mar. **https://www.acog.org/clinical/clinical-guidance/obstetric-care-consensus/articles/2020/03/management-of-stillbirth**
3. Zhang JT, Lee R, Sauer MV, Ananth CV. Risks of placental abruption and preterm delivery in patients undergoing assisted reproduction. JAMA Netw Open. 2024;7(7):e2420970. doi:10.1001/jamanetworkopen.2024.20970

INDEX

ABOUT THE AUTHOR

Jennifer Lincoln, MD, IBCLC, is a board-certified OB-GYN who practices clinically as an OB hospitalist, which is an obstetrician with expertise in handling obstetrical emergencies and making Labor and Delivery a safer place for all birthing patients. She has served as the president for the Society of OB/GYN Hospitalists, her specialty's national organization. She is also an International Board Certified Lactation Consultant (IBCLC). She is dedicated to developing evidence-based health content that is easy to understand and uses social media to educate millions of followers by meeting them where they are. Her voice is sought after in the reproductive health space, and she has been an invited guest in the White House and at the United Nations. She is married to a pediatrician, and together they have two boys and reside in Portland, Oregon.

ABOUT THE TYPE

This book was set in Caslon, a typeface first designed in 1722 by William Caslon (1692–1766). Its widespread use by most English printers in the early eighteenth century soon supplanted the Dutch typefaces that had formerly prevailed. The roman is considered a "workhorse" typeface due to its pleasant, open appearance, while the italic is exceedingly decorative.